T0198068

Pocket Reference to
Health Disorders

Pocket Reference to Health Disorders

Linda C. deWolfe Fritschle
Susan R. Rudnick

Rowman & Allanheld
Totowa, New Jersey

ROWMAN & ALLANHELD

Published in the United States of America in 1983
by Rowman & Allanheld
(A division of Littlefield, Adams & Company)
81 Adams Drive, Totowa, New Jersey 07512

Library of Congress Cataloging in Publication Data

Fritschle, Linda C. deWolfe, 1939-
  Pocket reference to health disorders.

  1. Pathology—Handbooks, manuals, etc.   I. Rudnick,
Susan R.   II. Title.
RB118.F73   1983   616.07'02'02   83-8692
ISBN 0-86598-126-4

83 84 85/10 9 8 7 6 5 4 3 2 1

Printed in the United States of America

Preface

As the number of health careers and health-related fields continues to grow, in response to the expansion of knowledge, technology, and public demand, there is an increasing need for a basic, concise reference book that can be used by those engaged in the many health-oriented disciplines.

This book is designed to provide concise descriptions of commonly found health conditions. Medical, surgical, mental, obstetric, and pediatric disorders and diseases are defined, symptomatology is described, and etiology, if known, is included. Selected terminology, applicable to mental disorders, has also been incorporated.

The purpose of this book is to offer concise reference information in a format that can be easily used. As a "pocket reference" this book is not intended to take the place of in-depth texts. It is our hope that the compact size of this book will enable the reader to use it in his or her own work or educational setting and that the content will serve as a stimulus for more in-depth reading.

The content has been organized alphabetically in order to facilitate referral. Entries have been cross-referenced where appropriate. Mental disorders have been entitled according to current classifications in the American Psychiatric Association's *Diagnostic and Statistical Manual,* 3d ed. (DSM III). Titles that were formerly in use have been cross-referenced to the currently accepted ones.

Acknowledgments

We wish to thank Mary Jo Aspinall, R.N., M.N., C.S., Series Editor, Rowman & Allanheld, Publishers, for inspiring us to write this book, thereby providing us with the opportunity to enhance our friendship and expand our knowledge.

We also wish to thank Mrs. C. L. deWolfe for her support and help in preparing drafts and preliminary work on the book, and the Rudnick family for their love, support, and patience.

Linda C. deWolfe Fritschle
Susan R. Rudnick

A

Aarskog Syndrome (faciogenital dysplasia). A hereditary X-linked condition characterized by shortness of stature, facial anomalies, and "saddle bag scrotum" (the scrotum overhangs the penis).

Abetalipoproteinemia (Bassen-Kornzweig syndrome, acanthocytosis). An inherited disorder (autosomal recessive trait) of lipid metabolism causing a decrease in lipid levels in plasma. Major clinical manifestations are malabsorption of fat, ataxia, muscular weakness and atrophy, retinitis pigmentosa, acanthocytosis, and a chronic progressive neurologic deficit usually beginning in childhood.

Abruptio Placentae (placental abruption, ablation placentae). During pregnancy, a premature detachment of the placenta from the wall of the uterus any time after the 20th week to the time of birth. Clinical findings include external hemorrhage of either bright or dark red blood, but the bleeding may be concealed and the uterus enlarges as the blood collects and infiltrates the muscle wall. Uterine tetany and tenderness, maternal hypotension, fetal death, and coagulopathy may be present.

Acanthocytosis. *See* Abetalipoproteinemia.

Achalasia. A motor disorder that involves the lower two-thirds portion of the esophagus. The esophageal sphincter pressure is elevated, there is no peristaltic response to swallowing, and relaxation of the sphincter is not complete. Symptoms can include substernal pain following eating, weight loss, dysphagia, and dilatation of the esophagus and stagnation of the food in the esophagus, often causing regurgitation.

Achondrogenesis. A congenital bone and connective tissue dysplasia characterized by low nasal bridge, short limbs, unmineralized vertebrae, and mental retardation.

Achondroplasia. A common type of dwarfism. A condition that is inherited (autosomal dominant trait). The length of the spine is usually normal but the limbs, hands, and feet are shortened. The head is large and accompanied by a saddle nose, and there is an exaggerated lumbar lordosis. There is normal mental and sexual development.

Acquired Immune Deficiency Syndrome (AIDS). A disease of unknown etiology, prominently affecting homosexual men, that causes a breakdown of the immune system. The result is often increased susceptibility to Kaposi's sarcoma and pulmonary infections.

Acrocephaly. A condition resulting from premature closure of the coronal suture of an infant. Clinical manifestations include exophthalmos, strabismus, nystagmus, papilledema, optic atrophy, and loss of vision.

Acrocyanosis. A benign vasospastic disorder that is characterized by persistent diffuse cyanosis of the fingers, hands, toes, and feet. The involved parts are usually cold and excessive perspiration is not uncommon.

Acrodynia (pink disease, Swift's disease, Feer's disease, erythredema, dermatopolyneuritis). A disease of infancy and early childhood resulting from mercury ingestion or contact. Clinical manifestations include listlessness, restlessness, irritability, rash, pink finger and toe tips, patchy areas of ischemia, edema and cyanosis of hands and feet, cold and clammy extremities, profuse perspiration, constant pain and pruritis in the hands and feet, dark necrotic nails, anorexia, photophobia, and peripheral neuritis.

Acrodysostosis. A congenital bone and connective tissue dysplasia characterized by low nasal bridge, maxillary hypoplasia, short hands and feet, short stature, and mental retardation.

Acromegaly. Pituitary growth hormone-secreting tumors, occurring after puberty, causing enlargement in the hands, feet, nose, and mandible, along with coarsening of facial features and a deep husky voice. Arthritis and limitation of joint motion may also be present.

Acroparesthesia. A sensory and motor paralysis (sleep palsy) (frequently occurring in adult women) caused by pressure of a nerve against an underlying bone during deep sleep. The patient is awakened with numbness, tingling, prickling, aching, and burning of the extremity. Vigorous rubbing usually restores normal sensation.

Addison's Disease. Adrenocortical hypofunction (primary adrenal insufficiency). Signs and symptoms include fatigability, weakness, anorexia, nausea and vomiting, weight loss, hypotension, hyperpigmentation, and abnormalities of GI function. Asthenia is the cardinal symptom.

Adenomyosis. A benign uterine disease characterized by infiltration of the myometrium with endometrial glands. Clinical manifestations include hypermenorrhea, dysmenorrhea, and a tender enlarged uterus.

Adie's Syndrome. A benign disorder of the parasympathetic innervation of the iris. The affected pupil is dilated and unreactive to light. Hyporeflexia, especially of knee jerks, is often also present.

Adjustment Disorder. A mental disorder that may occur at any age in response to a specific stressful event. Excessive responses to the event are commonly found and interpersonal relationships or work activities may be affected. Symptoms include anxiety, conduct disturbances, depressed mood, and social withdrawal. The disorder resolves with removal of the stressor or by the development of new coping mechanisms.

Adrenogenital Syndrome. An inherited condition in women resulting from an overproduction of androgens. Clinical features include masculinization, incomplete female development, clitoral hypertrophy, and amenorrhea.

Adrenoleukodystrophy. A hereditary metabolic disease of the nervous system (autosomal recessive). Signs and symptoms include dementia, decline in cognitive function, seizures, failing vision, cerebellar ataxia, and progressive polyneuropathy. Bronzing of the skin, homonymous hemianopsia, cortical blindness, hemiparesis, and aphasia may be present. Usual onset is in early childhood and the outcome is usually fatal.

Adult Respiratory Distress Syndrome (ARDS). A descriptive term used for many acute, diffusive infiltrative lung disorders that involve severe arterial hypoxemia. Clinical manifestations include tachypnea, dyspnea, rales, and cyanosis.

Adynamia Episodica Hereditaria (Gamstorp's Disease). A hereditary (mendelian dominant) condition characterized by periods of weakness or paralysis of skeletal muscle. Onset is between five and ten years of age. Weakness may last from one to several hours or up to weeks or months.

Affect. The overall feeling tone or emotional state of an individual conveyed by facial expressions, gestures, and tone of voice.

Affective Disorders. Mental disorders that are characterized by a depressed or elated mood. (Depression, Major; Bipolar Disorders; Cyclothymic Disorder; Dysthymic Disorder.)

Affective Syndrome, Organic. A mental condition caused by organic factors such as endocrine disorders or toxic substances. Symptoms correspond to either major depressive or manic episodes.

African Trypanosomiasis. *See* Sleeping Sickness.

Agonadism (the Absent Testes syndrome). A condition in which testicular growth failure occurred during gestation. Clinical syndromes vary from complete failure of virilization to incomplete virilization of external genitalia to normal males with bilateral anorchia.

Agnosia. An inability to identify sensations due to a disturbance in perception. Common objects, either viewed or touched, may not be recognized. The ability to identify familiar sounds may also be affected.

Agoraphobia. A phobic disorder characterized by an exceptional dread of being alone or in some public areas that leads to an increasing curtailment of activities. The need to continually avoid such situations may become the paramount influence in an individual's life.

Aicardi Syndrome. An inherited developmental condition characterized by seizures, corpus callosum defects, dorsal vertebral anomalies, mental retardation, large areas of chorioretinopathy, and microphthalmos.

AIDS. *See* Acquired Immune Deficiency Syndrome.

Albers-Schönberg Disease. An inherited osteopetrosis (marble bone disease) characterized by anemia, neurologic abnormalities, and pathologic fractures. Increased bone mass occurs and both bone formation and resorption are depressed. Cranial nerve abnormalities are often present and infections such as osteomyelitis are frequent.

Albinism. A hereditary (autosomal recessive) trait characterized by hypomelanosis of the skin and hair, photophobia, nystagmus, and translucent irides.

Albright's Hereditary Osteodystrophy (pseudohypoparathyroidism). An inherited condition characterized by the failure of the kidneys and the skeleton to respond to parathormone. Clinical manifestations include short, stocky stature, round face, growth failure, bradydactylia, skeletal abnormalities, and mental retardation.

Albright's Syndrome (fibrous dysplasia). Polyostotic fibrous dysplasia lesions, leading to skeletal deformities and/or fractures, are present. Abnormal cutaneous pigmentation (brown to light brown macules) tend to occur unilaterally. Sexual precocity of unknown cause is found in women.

Alcohol Abuse. A substance-use disorder characterized by daily consumption of alcohol, an inability to decrease or eliminate use despite efforts to stop, memory losses during drinking episodes, and prolonged periods of intoxication. Interpersonal relationships and/or work productivity are adversely affected by the pattern of use.

Alcohol Amnestic Disorder. A severely disabling and chronic organic mental disorder including short- and long-term memory loss caused by vitamin deficiency related to long-standing alcohol abuse. The routine administration of thiamine during detoxification has reduced the incidence of this disorder.

Alcohol Dependence (alcoholism). Includes characteristics of alcohol abuse. In addition, the dependent individual consumes increasingly larger amounts of alcohol in order to attain the needed effect and experiences physical withdrawal symptoms if consumption is reduced or eliminated.

Alcohol Intoxication. An organic mental disorder caused by and limited to recent alcohol consumption. Alterations in judgment and offensive or assaultive acts characterize the behaviors that impede the individual's ability to either relate to others or work. Accompanying signs include agitation, alterations in mood, decreased attention span, flushed face, poor coordination, and slurred speech.

Alcohol Withdrawal. An organic mental disorder resulting from either an abrupt reduction or elimination of alcohol consumption by an individual who has been alcohol dependent for many years. Symptoms appear within a few hours and include tremors accompanied by agitation, depressed mood, hypertension, nausea and vomiting, tachycardia, or weakness symptoms, usually resolving within one week.

Alcohol Withdrawal Delirium (delirium tremens). An organic mental disorder resulting from either an abrupt reduction or elimination of alcohol consumption by an individual who has been alcohol dependent for many years. Symptoms usually appear two to three days after the change in drinking pattern and are characterized by an altered state of consciousness with a decreased ability to respond to external stimuli. Delusions, hallucinations, and marked irritability are usually present and are accompanied by diaphoresis, hypertension, tachycardia, and tremors. Symptoms usually resolve within two to three days.

Alcoholism. *See* Alcohol Dependence.

Alcoholism, Dementia associated with. An organic mental disorder characterized by intellectual impairment resulting from long-term dependency on alcohol. Losses in abstract thinking, impulse control, judgment, and memory may be accompanied by changes in personality. Disability may range from very mild losses to an inability to maintain independent functioning.

Aldosteronism. A syndrome associated with hypersecretion from the adrenal glands of the hormone aldosterone. Primary—signifies that the problem is within the gland; secondary—the problem is of extraadrenal origin. Symptoms include potassium depletion, headaches associated with diastolic hypertension, muscle weakness and fatigue, polyuria, and polydipsia.

Alper's Disease. An inherited condition characterized by degeneration of gray matter of the brain in infancy. The prominent findings are seizures and dementia.

Alport's Syndrome. Sensorineural deafness associated with hereditary nephritis. Progressive but slow renal insufficiency terminates in end-stage renal disease associated with other abnormalities such as spherophakia, lenticonus, thrombocytopathia, hyperprolinemia, and cerebral dysfunction. Symptom of hematuria occurs at an early age.

Alzheimer's Disease. A progressive dementia with diffuse brain atrophy. Occurs during every age period but most often in later decades. Subtle onset with recent memory loss, depression, anxiety, and unpredictable behavioral quirks. In advanced stages a shuffling gait with muscle stiffness and awkwardness appear. CAT scan findings reveal enlargement of the ventricular system due to brain atrophy. The progression is gradual and steady and often terminates in total helplessness.

Amebiasis. An amoebic infection of the colon. Foul-smelling, chronic mild diarrhea to fulminating bloody dysentery can occur, but most patients are asymptomatic carriers. Hepatic abscess can be a complication and can rupture into the peritoneum, pleura, lung, or pericardium.

Amnesia, Psychogenic. *See* Psychogenic Amnesia and Fugue.

Amnestic Syndrome. A mental condition caused by organic factors such as head trauma, hypoxia, or thiamine deficiency. It is characterized by short- and long-term memory loss. The loss is usually not recognized by the individual who may use confabulation to compensate for lapses in memory. The condition may be both chronic and severely incapacitating.

Amphetamine Abuse and Dependence. ABUSE is characterized by almost daily use and an inability to decrease or eliminate use, which may result in delusional episodes or clouding of consciousness (*see* Amphetamine Organic Mental Disorders). Interpersonal relationships and/or work productivity are adversely affected by the pattern of use.

DEPENDENCE is evidenced by the need for increasingly larger amounts of the substance in order to attain the needed effect and by the individual experiencing withdrawal symptoms if intake is decreased or eliminated.

Amphetamine Organic Mental Disorders. Intoxication adversely affects judgment, interpersonal relationships, and/or work productivity and is manifested within one hour of use by symptoms that include elation, grandiosity, nausea and vomiting, psychomotor agitation, pupillary dilation, and tachycardia. DELIRIUM, consisting of clouding of consciousness and perceptual disturbances, may also occur within one hour of drug use and last for about six hours with long-term usage. A DELUSIONAL SYNDROME may develop. Persecutory delusions are characteristic and may be accompanied by aggressiveness, ideas of reference, and psychomotor agitation. The disorder may persist for over a year. Withdrawal from amphetamines after long-term use develops within a few days of decreasing or eliminating use and peaks within two to four days. Symptoms include depressed mood, fatigue, and sleep disturbances.

Amyloidosis. An extracellular fibrous protein amyloid disposition in sites throughout the body. Liver, kidney, spleen, and heart enlargement may become evident. Clinical symptoms depend upon the area of body involvement. Generalized, the condition usually ends in death after several years.

Amyotrophic Lateral Sclerosis. A progressive motor neuron (in the cerebral cortex, brainstem, and spinal cord) degenerative disease. Symptoms include spasticity with tendon reflex exaggeration, muscular weakness and atrophy, and hyperreflexia. Progression is rapid and may lead to death in two to five years from respiratory muscle paralysis.

Anencephaly. A congenital anomaly characterized by absence of the membranous skull and cerebral hemispheres. Infants are either stillborn or die within a few days.

Angioimmunoblastic Lymphadenopathy with Dysprotein-emia (AILD). A systemic disorder presenting with hepatomegaly, splenomegaly, and lymphadenopathy. Clinical manifestations include fever, weight loss, pruritis, and skin rashes. This disorder is considered to be a severe hypersensitivity reaction.

Ankloglossia. *See* Tongue-Tie.

Ankylosing Spondylitis. (Marie-Strumpell disease). A chronic and progressive inflammatory process (of unknown etiology) affecting sacroiliac, hip, shoulder, and peripheral joints. Usually affects thirty-year-old men. Symptoms include pain in hips, shoulders, and buttocks, and anterior chest pain. Advanced stages present with a bent posture, rigid spine, dorsal kyphosis, and abnormal gait. Treatment is aimed at prevention of deformities.

Anorexia Nervosa (Twiggy syndrome). A condition mostly seen in females of prepuberty to mid-life, characterized by self-induced starvation and emaciation but without associated lethargy. Amenorrhea, physical overactivity, self-induced vomiting, hypotension, and constipation with excessive use of laxatives are all clinical manifestations. Emotionally the patient is usually an intelligent perfectionist who is obsessed with fear of obesity.

Anthrax (Woolsorter's disease). A disease transmitted to man by contact with infected animals or their products. The main lesion is the malignant pustule (a necrotic ulcer) accompanied by extensive edema. Widespread infection with mediastinitis may also occur. The disease can be local and mild to disseminated and rapidly fatal.

Antisocial Personality Disorder. A personality disorder characterized by ongoing patterns of behavior that include the inability to develop or maintain lasting relationships and the violation of accepted legal or moral responsibilities by the individual, who will lie to and manipulate others in order to achieve goals. There is a long-standing pattern of superficial interpersonal relationships, frequent job changes and unemployment, aggressiveness, and impulsivity. The disorder is manifested by adolescence and continues into adulthood. Previously, individuals with this disorder have been referred to as psychopaths or sociopaths.

Anxiety. A sensation of diffuse discomfort or apprehension resulting from a perceived threat to the self, the source of which is not clearly defined.

Anxiety Disorder, Generalized. A mental disorder in which continued, generalized anxiety is experienced. Manifestations include agitation, apprehension, autonomic hyperactivity, restlessness, trembling, sleep disturbances, and continual worrying.

Anxiety Disorders. A group of mental disorders in which symptoms of anxiety are a prominent feature. These include generalized anxiety, panic, phobia, and obsessive compulsive disorders.

Anxiety Neuroses. *See* Anxiety Disorder, Generalized; Panic Disorder.

Aortic Septal Defect (aortopulmonary septal defect). A congenital cardiovascular lesion in which there is an opening between the aorta and the pulmonary artery above the semilunar valves. Left to right shunting of blood occurs, accompanied by obstructive pulmonary disease and pulmonary arterial hypertension.

Aortic Sinus Aneurysm and Fistula. A congenital progressive aneurysmal dilatation of an aortic sinus of Valsalva. It may rupture into the cardiac chamber (usually the right ventricle) forming an aorticocardiac fistula. Rupture causes chest pain, constant arteriovenous shunting, and bilateral ventricular volume overload with heart failure.

Apert Syndrome (acrocephalosyndactyly). An inherited condition characterized by pointing of the head anteriorly and syndactyly of the hands and feet.

Appendicitis. An inflammation of the lumen of the appendix due to bacterial infection, obstruction, parasites, or lymphoid hyperplasia. Clinical manifestations include localized right lower quadrant pain, rebound tenderness, nausea and vomiting, anorexia, and indigestion.

Apraxia. The loss of ability to perform specific purposeful movements without loss of motor function or sensation.

Arachnodactyly. *See* Marfan Syndrome.

Arrhenoblastoma (Sertoli-Leydig cell tumor). An androgen-secreting ovarian tumor producing virilization. Clinical manifestations include oligomenorrhea, breast tissue atrophy, hirsutism, clitoromegaly, hoarseness, alopecia, and adnexal mass.

Arteriosclerosis. A thickening and hardening of the arterial wall caused by an accumulation of smooth muscle cells and connective tissue in the intima along with spingomyelin and cholesterol linoleate. Vessels become rigid, arteries dilate and elongate, and aneurysms may form in the "plaque."

Articulation Disorder, Developmental. A disorder found in children who, despite normal hearing and language development, are unable to consistently pronounce some later acquired sounds, such as *ch, f, l, r,* or *sh.*

Asbestosis. An environmental lung disease that develops into diffuse pulmonary fibrosis slowly after a long latent period following exposure to asbestos inhalation. Dyspnea, basal rales, and decreased vital capacity occur. Cigarette smoke and asbestos interact as causative factors of lung cancer.

Ascariasis. A worm infection (ascaris lumbricoides) resulting in a lung infestation and later in intestinal infiltration. Bronchopneumonia may occur as the larvae pass through the lungs. Intestinal symptoms may include abdominal pain, vomiting, or passing the worms in the stool. Complications such as volvulus, intussusception, and intestinal obstruction are possible.

Ask-Upmark Syndrome (segmental hypoplasia). A renal condition characterized by a reduction in the number of renal lobules with arrest in development in one or more. The main clinical problem is hypertension, which usually occurs at ten years of age.

Asthma. An airway passage disease. Air passages narrow (usually in response to stimuli or an external irritant). Dyspnea, cough, and sneezing are clinically evident. Edema of the bronchial wall and thick tenacious secretions occur. As airway passage diameter is reduced, increased airway resistance results in decreased expiratory flow, hyperinflation of the lungs and thorax, and abnormal distribution of pulmonary blood flow.

Astrocytoma. A slow-growing infiltrative tumor of the brain or spinal cord, the majority of which undergo malignant degeneration. Convulsions, headache, giddiness, vomiting, dull and stuporous states, and psychic changes are presenting symptoms.

Asymmetric Septal Hypertrophy. *See* Idiopathic Hypertrophic Subaortic Stenosis.

Atelectasis. Collapse of pulmonary alveoli caused by mucus, mecomium, or foreign body obstruction. Clinical manifestations include fever, tachypnea, decreased breath sounds, rales, and dyspnea.

Atherosclerosis. A type of arteriosclerosis involving primarily the intimal layer of the vessel and occurring mostly in the abdominal aorta, renal branches, coronary arteries, and cerebral vessels. It is characterized by focal discrete raised fibromuscular plaques. Lesions are irregularly distributed.

Athlete's Foot. *See* Dermatophytosis.

Atrial Septal Defect. A congenital cardiac condition manifested by patency of the atrial septum allowing oxygenated blood to shunt from the left atrium of the heart into the right. Diastolic overload of the right ventricle and in-

creased pulmonary blood flow occur. Usually asymptomatic in early life; after forty, atrial arrhythmias and
pulmonary atrial hypertension develop and cardiac failure
results.

Attention Deficit Disorder. A disorder that is found in
children before the age of seven, more commonly in boys.
It is characterized by impulsiveness and a lack of attention
that is not in accord with the child's stage of development.
Manifestations include difficulty in organizing and com-
pleting tasks, carelessness, difficulty in following instruc-
tions and in concentrating, and an increased need for
supervision. Some children with this disorder are also
hyperactive and may exhibit difficulty sitting still,
restlessness, and excessive running.

Autism, Infantile. *See* Infantile Autism.

Avellis Syndrome. A brainstem disorder (usually caused by a
tumor) involving the tenth cranial nerve. Paralysis of vocal
cords and soft palate occur along with contralateral
hemiplegia.

Avoidant Personality Disorder. A personality disorder characterized by long-standing patterns of behavior that severely impede the development of meaningful interpersonal
relationships. Individuals with this disorder exhibit low
self-esteem and are unwilling to enter into relationships due
to an exaggerated fear of rejection. Despite the need
for interpersonal closeness, they withdraw from such op-
portunities unless they receive prior commitments of
acceptance.

B

Babesiosis. A protozoan infection of animals, transmitted to man by ticks, producing acute febrile illness. Hemolytic anemia and hemoglobinuria occur. At present there are no available drugs for treatment. Infestation can be self-limited or life-threatening.

Baker's Cysts. Cysts of the popliteal fossa. Cause unknown, but trauma can be a stimulant to formation. If cyst ruptures, acute extensive inflammation, swelling, and pain of the lower leg results. Unruptured cysts cause aching and pain in the leg.

Balantidiasis. A protozoan infestation of the large intestine producing a carrier state or disease ranging from mild recurring diarrhea to fulminating ulceration, performation, and death. More prevalent in tropical areas. Swine and rats are common carriers.

Banti's Syndrome. Chronic congestive splenomegaly characterized by splenomegaly, pancytopenia, portal hypertension, and GI bleeding. Caused by portal hypertension due to intra- or extrahepatic pathology. Prognosis is determined by underlying cause.

Barbiturate Abuse and Dependence. ABUSE is evidenced by an individual who is intoxicated for a major portion of the day, experiences memory losses while intoxicated, and who is not able to either reduce or eliminate use. DEPEND-ENCE includes the characteristics of abuse, but also involves the need to take increasingly larger amounts in order to attain the needed effects, or by the experiencing of withdrawal symptoms if use is decreased or eliminated.

Barbiturate Organic Mental Disorders. There are four or-

ganic disorders related to barbiturate use. INTOXICA-
TION is manifested shortly after use by symptoms that include irritability, mood swings, impaired judgment, slurred
speech, poor coordination, and decreased attention span.
An AMNESTIC DISORDER, characterized by short- and
long-term memory loss, may be caused by long-standing
heavy use. WITHDRAWAL, experienced after a decrease
in amount or elimination of the drug after long-standing
and/or heavy use, may result in symptoms that include
restlessness, nausea and vomiting, tremors, autonomic
hyperactivity, and weakness. A WITHDRAWAL DELIR-
IUM may occur within a week of a decrease or elimination
of heavy use. Symptoms include autonomic hyperactivity,
sleep and perceptual disturbances, disorientation, and
clouding of consciousness.

Bardet-Biedl Syndrome. *See* Biedl-Bardet Syndrome.

Barlow's Syndrome. *See* Systolic Click-Murmur Syndrome.

Bartholin Duct Cyst. A vaginal cyst arising in the duct system
of the Bartholin gland as a result of obstruction of the duct.
Abscess forms when the cyst becomes infected. Clinically
the patient presents with pain and tenderness over the infected gland, edema of the labia, and inflammation of skin.

Bartonellosis (Carrion's disease). A bacterial infection with
two clinical stages: a rapid-onset, acute febrile anemia
(Oroya fever), and a benign stage manifesting chronic
eruptive cutaneous lesions (verruga peruana). The first
stage carries a high mortality rate. Extreme pallor,
weakness and drop in red blood cell count occur. Asymptomatic "carrier" cases can also occur.

Bartter's Syndrome. An inherited functional renal tubular
defect resulting in chronic potassium depletion, excessive
production of PGE, and elevated concentration of
angiotension II. Symptoms include weakness, periodic
paralysis, and polyuria. Excessive salt and water lost in the
urine result in extracellular fluid volume depletion. Blood
pressure remains normal.

Basedow's Disease. *See* Grave's disease.

Bassen-Kornzweig Syndrome. *See* Abetalipoproteinemia.

Batten-Spielmeyer-Vogt Lipidosis. An inherited degenerative disorder characterized by derangement of lipid metabolism causing lipid accumulation in nervous system and organ cells. Death of affected nervous cell eventually occurs. Onset is between five to ten years of age and progression ends with early adulthood death. Symptoms include visual impairment, cerebellar ataxia, and dementia. This type of liposis is not confined to Jewish people.

Beal Syndrome. A genetic condition characterized by long fused ear lobes, radial-head, elbow dysplasia, long prominent scapulae, and short stature.

Becker Pseudohypertrophic Muscular Dystrophy. A sex-linked genetic mild form of muscular dystrophy. Muscle weakness is not severe and walking is possible in most patients. Cardiologic changes are not frequent. Creatine phosphokinase serum levels are elevated although not high.

Beckwith's Syndrome. A congenital abnormality characterized by excessive birth size in association with umbilical abnormalities, macroglossia, renal enlargement, microcephaly, and facial flame nevus.

Behçet's Syndrome. A syndrome of unknown etiology manifested by oral and genital ulcers and ocular inflammation. Arthritis, thrombophlebitis, neurological abnormalities, fever, colitis, and skin lesions may also be present. These clinical manifestations are caused by vasculitis of small- and medium-sized vessels. The clinical course is variable with exacerbations occurring in weeks, months, or years. Mortality is high when central nervous system involvement is present.

Behr Syndrome. An inherited condition characterized by optic atrophy, ataxia and loss of coordination, mental deficiency, pyramidal tract signs, and vesical sphincter weakness.

Bell's Palsy. A temporary facial paralysis of newborn babies usually associated with forcep delivery. Clinical features include closure of the eyelid on the affected side and distortion of the mouth toward the unaffected side.

Benedikt's Syndrome. A brainstem disorder (caused by a tumor, hemorrhage, tuberculoma, or softening) affecting the third cranial nerve. Oculomotor palsy with contralateral cerebellar ataxia, tremor, and corticospinal signs occur.

Berger's Disease (idiopathic renal hematuria). A disease characterized by recurrent hematuria. Prominent IgA deposits found in the mesangium confirm the diagnosis. Hematuria can be associated with flulike illness or vigorous exercise. The disease progresses slowly and end-stage renal failure can occur in approximately twenty-five years.

Beriberi. A disease of thiamine deficiency consisting of two major syndromes: 1. cardiovascular (wet beriberi) manifested by such problems as peripheral vasodilatation, tachycardia, increased cardiac output, and venous congestion with sodium retention and edema; and 2. nervous systems (dry beriberi). Three types of nervous systems have been identified: 1. peripheral neuropathy manifested by loss of sensory, motor and reflex function; 2. Wernicke's encephalopathy (cerebral beriberi) manifested by vomiting, nystagmus, fever, ataxia and mental deterioration; and 3. Korsakoff's syndrome manifested by retrograde amnesia and impaired ability to learn. Most patients with beriberi have a mixture of the syndromes.

Bezoars. A conglomerate of food and mucus or vegetable matter that has formed in the gastric remnant following partial gastrectomy. Symptoms include anorexia, epigastric fullness, nausea, and vomiting. Removal can often be accomplished with gastric lavage.

Bezold's Abscess. A suppuration on the submastoid space, usually secondary to otitis. It produces nuchal rigidity. The infection sometimes extends down the carotid sheath to the mediastinum.

Biedl-Bardet Syndrome (Laurence-Moon-Biedl [LMB] syndrome). A hereditary condition manifested by obesity, digital anomalies, hypogonadism, retinal degeneration, and mental retardation. Severe kidney abnormalities may also be present as well as cardiac anomalies.

Bielschowsky Syndrome. An inherited condition characterized by degeneration with onset between the ages of one to three years. Clinical manifestations include progressive loss of vision, seizures, hyperactivity, irritability, speech deterioration, cerebellar ataxia, tremor, rigidity, spastic paralysis, and dementia.

Biglieri's Syndrome. A 17 $\propto$ hydroxylase enzymatic deficiency disorder resulting in impairment of ovarian and adenocortical function. The disorder appears in young women manifesting sexual infantilism with elevated gonadotrophin levels and hypertension. Sex steroids and corticosteroids replacement therapy is usually indicated.

Bilharziasis. *See* Schistosomiasis.

Bipolar Disorder, Depressed. An affective disorder diagnosed when an individual who has previously had one or more manic episodes evidences symptoms of a major depression.

Bipolar Disorder, Manic. An affective mental disorder characterized by the occurrence of manic episodes that are distinct periods of time in which symptoms of the disorder are manifested. Many individuals are symptom-free between episodes. The episodes are characterized by a mood that is elevated or expansive, increased activity levels, flight of ideas, pressured speech, irritability, inflated self-esteem, decreased appetite, and a decreased need for sleep. Mood swings are common and delusions or hallucinations may be present. Dress may be inappropriate or bizarre, and activities such as buying sprees and grandiose business ventures may be undertaken.

Bipolar Disorder, Mixed. An affective mental disorder diagnosed when an individual evidences symptoms of both a manic episode and a major depressive episode. The symp-

toms may alternate every few days or they may be inter-
mixed. The depressive features are most pronounced.

Blackwater Fever. A disorder of unknown cause that ac-
companies *P. falciparum* malaria. The onset begins with
rigor and fever. Massive intravascular hemolysis, icterus,
hemoglobinuria, and acute renal failure follow. Mortality
occurs in 30 percent of the cases.

Blastomycosis (Gilchrist's disease). A fungal infection presenting as chronic pneumonia and/or chronic skin eruptions. Inhalation of the fungus from the air seems to be the
cause. The infection can also spread to subcutaneous tissue
and bones. The presenting clinical manifestations include
cough, weight loss, malaise, skin lesions, chest pain, and
fever.

Bloom Syndrome. An inherited dermatosis characterized by
erythema of the face, photosensitivity, small stature, and
low birth weight.

Blount's Disease. An acquired bone lesion of the proximal
tibial metaphysis and epiphysis of unknown cause. The
result is bowleggedness.

Bolivian Hemorrhagic Fever. A viral infection transmitted by
the urine of *C. callosus* (a mouselike rodent). Clinical
manifestations include fever, dehydration, hypotension,
oliguria, and bradycardia. Bleeding from gums, hematemesis, hematuria, and melena occur in severe cases.
Shock, hypothermia, GI bleeding, and pulmonary edema
may precede death. Mortality rate can be as high as 30
percent.

Bonnevie-Ullrich Syndrome. *See* Gonadal Dygenesis.

Borderline Personality Disorder. A personality disorder characterized by long-standing patterns of behavior that may
seriously impede interpersonal relationships and employment. Manifestations include impulsiveness, limited ability
to control anger, persistent feelings of emptiness, and mood

swings. Both the individual's self-image and interpersonal relationships are typified by their instability.

Borderline Schizophrenia. *See* Schizotypal Personality Disorder.

Bornholm's Disease (pleurodynia, epidemic myalgia). A viral infection causing malaise, sore throat, anorexia, fever, and pleuritic and abdominal muscle pain. The duration is three to seven days, but relapses can occur. Meningitis, myocarditis, and hepatitis can ensue. Orchitis may also develop.

Botulism. An acute form of food poisoning caused by ingesting foods contaminated with *Clostridium botulinum*. It is the toxin of the organism that produces muscle paralysis and fatality. Disease can be mild to fulminating. Symptoms usually begin from twelve to thirty-six hours after ingestion and include visual disturbances, weakness of the tongue, paralysis of extremities, nausea and vomiting, constipation, and decreased salivation. The biggest threat is respiratory failure.

Bourneville's Disease (tuberous sclerosis). An inherited disease manifesting convulsive seizures, mental deficiency, and adenoma sebaceum (fine wartlike lesions appearing on the cheeks and forehead). Retinal tumors, spina bifida, cataracts, and other malformations may be present. Death usually occurs before age thirty.

Bowen's Disease. A squamous cell carcinoma of the skin. Exposure to arsenic is one of the predominant causes. Skin lesions are finely defined thickened plaques that are brownish-red in color. Lesions are easily treatable by surgery. This condition is associated with an increased risk of visceral carcinomas.

Brachial Muscular Dystrophy. *See* Syringomelic Syndrome.

Brachial Plexus Injury (Erb's or Duchenne's palsy). A birth injury to the lower cervical and upper thoracic nerve root usually caused by lateral traction of the head or downward traction on the shoulder and arm of the infant during delivery. Varying degrees of arm paralysis result, which may resolve or are permanent.

Brenner Tumor. An ovarian neoplasm that is benign. Clinical manifestations include abdominal enlargement, pain, and menstrual irregularities.

Brief Reactive Psychosis. A psychotic disorder lasting less than two weeks that is characterized by a sudden onset after an unusually stressful event. Symptoms include delusions, hallucinations, loosening of associations, and disorganized behavior.

Broca's Aphasia (motor aphasia). A syndrome manifesting failure of the motor aspects of speaking and writing. The patient has trouble speaking aloud. The lower face on the right sags and the tongue deviates also to that side. Weakness in the right arm and leg are also present. Frontal lobe tumor or abscess or infection due to occlusion of the left middle cerebral artery is usually the cause.

Brodie's Abscess. A staphylococcal infection localized within the dense granulation tissue of bone. It remains about a central necrotic cavity and can persist for years.

Bronchiectasis. An irreversible dilatation of the large bronchi because of destruction of the elasticity and muscle in the bronchial wall. Causes can be bacterial infection, genetic, or mechanical. The symptoms include chronic cough with sputum production, hemoptysis, and recurrent pneumonia.

Bronchitis. Chronic bronchitis is an illness manifesting excessive tracheobronchial mucus production. It is associated with hyperplasia and hypertrophy of the mucus-producing glands. Contributing factors are cigarette smoking, air pollution, infection, and genetic factors.

Bronze Baby Syndrome. A condition caused by phototherapy treatment, characterized by a dark, grayish-brown skin discoloration. Hyperbilirubinemia is present and may last for months.

Brucellosis (undulant fever). A disease that is caused by an organism transmitted to man from goats, swine, cattle, or sheep. Spread may be airborne, through cow's milk, or by dermal contact. Incubation period is five to twenty-one days. Onset may be insidious with symptoms of low-grade fever, headache, insomnia, anorexia, and generalized aches and pains. Other symptoms include pain over the spine and pain along peripheral nerves. Orchitis is common. Bedrest usually results in prompt improvement. Permanent remission is usual within three to six months, although in some patients the disease may persist for years.

Bruton's Disease. A congenital agammaglobulinemia. Clinical manifestations usually appear at two years of age and consist of severe recurrent infections and rheumatoidlike arthritis.

Bubbly-Lung Syndrome (Wilson-Mikity syndrome, bronchopulmonary dysplasia). A condition of unknown etiology occurring in premature infants of less than 1500 grams. Clinical manifestations include dyspnea, tachypnea, retractions, and cyanosis. Complications include pneumonitis, collapse of a lung, and right heart failure.

Buerger-Crutz Syndrome. An inherited hyperlipoproteinemia. Clinical manifestations include bouts of abdominal pain and vomiting.

Bulimia. A mental disorder characterized by recurrent episodes of binge eating and fasting. The individual is aware that eating habits are not normal but is afraid of not being able to control the amount of food intake. It occurs more frequently in females, usually starting during adolescence or early adulthood.

Bursitis. An inflammation of any of the bursae between tendons, muscles, and bony prominences, the most common site being the shoulder, with acute onset. The pain may be severe especially with any rotation or abduction of joints. In chronic cases the pain is intermittent and nagging.

Byssinosis. A respiratory illness occurring among cotton textile workers and caused by chemical agents in textile ducts. Symptoms include cough, wheezing, and chest tightness. After ten to twenty years of exposure, severe airway obstruction and diminished elastic recoil of the lungs occur.

C

Caffeine Intoxication (caffeinism). An organic disorder caused by recent intake of caffeine. Effects may be evidenced by intake of as little as 250 mg. of caffeine by some individuals (one cup of coffee has 150 mg. of caffeine). Effects include diuresis, gastrointestinal disturbances, excitement, flushed face, insomnia, and restlessness.

California (LaCrosse) Encephalitis. A viral infection of squirrels carried to man by mosquitoes. Two clinical patterns have been defined: a mild form with two to three days of fever, headache, malaise, and GI symptoms followed by lethargy and meningeal signs abating in seven to eight days; and a severe form with fever, headache and vomiting followed by lethargy, disorientation, seizures, focal neurological signs, and coma.

Camurati-Engelmann Syndrome. An inherited developmental disorder characterized by thickening of the cortices of the long bones and neuromuscular dystrophy. There is wasting of the muscles and a characteristic waddling gait.

Canavan's Disease. An inherited spongy degeneration of the cerebral white matter terminating in death usually by age five. Clinical manifestations include blindness, poor head control, rigidity, hyperreflexia, and progressive macrocephaly.

Cancer. A term signifying abnormal cell growth that may result in the invasion of normal tissue and/or spread to other organs (metastasis).

Candidiasis. A yeastlike fungal infection. Infection of the oral-pharyngeal and vaginal mucosa is called thrush and is manifested by adhering white plaques and fissuring at the mouth corners. The cutaneous infection presents as red macerated intertriginous areas. Chronic mucocutaneous infection has typical hyperkeratotic skin lesions, crumbling nails, partial alopecia, and both oral and vaginal thrush. Persons who have diabetes mellitus or who are being treated with broad spectrum antibiotics are particularly susceptible.

Cannabis Abuse and Dependence. ABUSE is manifested by almost daily use of cannabis, extended periods of intoxication, and delusional episodes. There is a resulting loss of interest in friends, work, and usual activities. In addition to the above, DEPENDENCE is characterized by the need for increasingly larger amounts of cannabis to maintain the same effects.

Cannabis Organic Mental Disorders. These include Cannabis intoxication and Cannabis delusional disorder. INTOXICATION is manifested shortly after use by tachycardia, which may be accompanied by apathy, euphoria, and a sense of time passing more slowly than usual. The individual may have an increased appetite, dry mouth, and demonstrate excessive anxiety, poor judgment, or paranoid ideation. A DELUSIONAL DISORDER is manifested by delusions that occur shortly after use. The delusions last a few hours, the usual duration of intoxication.

Capillariasis, Intestinal. A round worm infestation resulting in intractable diarrhea with a high mortality rate. There is an accompanying malabsorption of fats and sugars and a protein-losing pathology. Hypokalemia, hypocalcemia, and hypoproteinemia occur as adult worms invade the small intestinal mucosa. Initially abdominal pain and intestinal gurgling occur followed by a copious watery diarrhea, anorexia, vomiting, weight loss, muscle wasting, weakness, hyporeflexia, and edema. Fluid and electrolyte replacement as well as medication causes dramatic improvement.

Cardiac Tamponade. A rapid filling of the pericardial space by fluid or blood resulting in pericardial effusion. The pressure on the heart interferes with diastolic filling of the ventricles and results in diminished cardiac output and circulatory failure. Clinical manifestations include distended neck veins, diminished heart tones, pulsus paradoxicus, dyspnea, cyanosis, and shock.

Carotenemia. A condition resulting from excessive ingestion of carotene-containing foods, mainly carrots. The condition is not harmful and does not lead to hypervitaminosis A. The condition is characterized by yellowing of the skin, mostly the palms of the hands and soles of the feet. The scleras remain white, but there is a yellowness of the serum.

Carpal Tunnel Syndrome (entrapment neuropathy). A condition caused by pressure on the median nerve as it passes through the space formed by the wrist bone and the transverse carpal ligament. Symptoms include numbness of the palmar surfaces of the first three digits of the hand, a weakened thumb adduction, and atrophy of the thenar eminence. Dryness of the skin in the area is also common.

Carpenter Syndrome. A congenital condition characterized by acrocephaly, peculiar facies, bradysyndactyly of the fingers, syndactyly of the toes, hypogenitalism, obesity, and mental retardation.

Carrión's Disease. *See* Bartonellosis.

Cataract. A gradually developing opacity of the lens or lens capsule commonly occurring bilaterally and resulting in vision loss. Clinical manifestations include seeing halos around lights, blinding glare from lights, poor reading vision, glare and poor vision in bright sunlight, and gradual blurring and loss of vision.

Catatonic Behavior. Motor activities characteristic of catatonic schizophrenia. These include excitement that is marked by agitated, sometimes violent, purposeless motor activity, negativism, posturing in which the individual may assume bizarre and uncomfortable positions, rigidity, stupor, and waxy flexibility in which an individual's limbs will maintain the position that they are placed in regardless of any discomfort.

Catatonic Type, Schizophrenic Disorders. *See* Schizophrenic Disorders, Catatonic Type.

Cat-Bite Fever. *See* Cat-Scratch Disease.

Cat-Cry Syndrome (Cri-du-chat). A genetic defect resulting in an infant with characteristic moon face, microcephaly, and severe mental retardation. The characteristic symptom is a weak, high-pitched cry resembling a cat's cry.

Cat-Eye Syndrome. An inherited condition characterized by microphthalmia, colomba, absent macular areas, anal atresia, preauricular skin tags, and umbilical hernia.

Cat-Scratch Disease. An infection resulting from a cat scratch. Manifestations include regional lymphadenitis. Splinters, thorns, dog, and monkey scratches can also cause the infection. Incubation period is three to ten days. Adenopathy can last as long as six weeks and is unilateral and symmetrical. Occasionally the nodes suppurate, soften, and drain. Other symptoms include headache, fever, and malaise.

Celiac Disease. A disorder of malabsorption, abnormal small intestine structure, and intolerance to glutten (wheat protein). Clinical manifestations include weight loss, abdominal distention, diarrhea, and steatorrhea. Bone pain and tenderness caused by demineralization of the bones are not uncommon. Emotional disturbances can also occur. A glutten-free diet results in improvement for most patients.

Cellulitis. An invasive infection of connective tissue resulting in reddish-brown discoloration and edema of the skin over the infected area and a moderate to high fever.

Cerebelloretinal Hemangioblastomatosis. *See* von Hippel-Lindau Syndrome.

Cerebral Palsy. A popular term for conditions of major disturbance of motor function, nonprogressive, with onset at an early age and of varying etiologic and characteristic factors. The pattern of paralysis or rigidity is important in order to ascertain cause and pathogenic mechanisms. The two etiologic mechanisms associated with this condition are prematurity and brain injury during birth. Clinical manifestations include paralysis (paraplegia, diplegia, and pseudobulbar) seizures, stiff awkward movements of legs, retarded development, speech difficulties, and ataxia.

Cestode Infections. Tapeworms attach to the host's intestinal mucosa releasing eggs as they mature. Most cases of the disease are asymptomatic but epigastric pain, diarrhea, weight loss, irritability, nausea, and an increase in appetite can occur. Movements of the worms may be apparent at the anus.

Chagas' Disease. A trypanosomiasis infection. Clinical manifestations include a local inflammatory reaction (erythematous nodule or chagoma) at the site of entry of the protozoan (usually the conjunctiva). This may persist for one to two months. As the protozoa infest the blood stream, fever, lymphadenopathy, hepatosplenomegaly, and edema of face and trunk appear. Myocarditis and severe heart disease are not uncommon.

Charcot-Marie-Tooth Disease. An inherited peroneal muscular atrophy usually appearing in late childhood. Clinical characteristics include foot drop, pes cavus, and peroneal myatrophy. The child has a "stork-leg" appearance and a high-steppage gait.

Chemodectoma. *See* Pheochromocytoma.

Chickenpox. A contagious viral disease transmitted by the respiratory route. Clinical manifestations appear ten to twenty-one days after exposure and include fever, malaise, and a pruritic maculopapular rash with lesions in all stages of development.

Cholecystitis. Inflammation of the gallbladder, usually caused by obstruction of the cystic duct by a calculus (gallstone). Symptoms include right upper quadrant abdominal pain worsened by respiration, nausea, and low-grade fever.

Choledocholithiasis (gallstones). They may be present without manifesting symptoms or they may accompany biliary colic, cholangitis (inflammation of the bile duct), and pancreatitis. Symptoms would then occur such as spiking fever, chills, colic, and jaundice. Pruritis and coagulopathy may be present if biliary cirrhosis develops. Septicemia and shock can occur.

Cholera. A bacterial-caused disease resulting in copious diarrhea and fluid and electrolyte depletion. Incubation period is six to forty-eight hours. Clinical manifestations include abrupt onset of watery painless ricelike diarrhea, vomiting, muscle cramps, cyanosis, poor skin turgor, thready tachycardia, high-pitched voice, and hypotension. The disease runs its course in two to seven days and with fluid and electrolyte replacement, recovery is usually complete.

Christmas Disease. A congenital bleeding disorder in which there is a deficiency in blood clotting factor IX. Clinically it manifests itself the same as hemophelia.

Chromomycosis. A skin condition caused by fungi and manifested by chronic verrucoid, ulcerated, or crusted skin lesions. Lesions are usually on feet and legs and begin as pimples, pustules, or ulcers, but slowly worsen over the years. Itching is common.

Chronic Motor Tic Disorder. *See* Tic Disorder, Chronic Motor.

Circumstantiality. Describes speech that is indirect and full of irrelevant facts and deficits, making it difficult to determine what ideas the individual is attempting to express.

Cirrhosis. A term that includes all types of chronic diffuse liver disease. Progressive reduction of liver cell mass is present resulting in jaundice, ascites, edema, central nervous system dysfunction, and cachexia. Portal venous hypertension with resultant esophageal and gastric varices and splenomegaly is not uncommon. Most types of cirrhosis can be attributed to alcoholic, postnecrotic, biliary, hemochromatosis, or cardiogenic causes.

Clanging. A pathological speech pattern that is characterized by the use of sounds such as rhymes and puns to determine choice of words rather than the idea to be expressed.

Clap. *See* Gonorrhea.

Claude's Syndrome. A brainstem syndrome involving the third cranial nerve and manifesting oculomotor palsy with contralateral cerebellar ataxia and tremor. Vascular occlusion, tumor, or aneurysm can be the cause.

Clonorchiasis. An infection of the biliary passages caused by the liver fluke. Can be asymptomatic unless worms cause biliary obstruction in which case fever, chills, tender hepatomegaly, and jaundice occur.

Coagulation, Disseminated Intravascular (DIC). A complex disorder usually occurring along with shock, sepsis, dissecting aneurysm of the aorta, massive venous thrombosis or pulmonary embolism. Bleeding from multiple sites, purpura, and ecchymosis are present. Fibrinogen is usually low and fibrinogen degradation products are usually high in the blood.

Coal Workers Pneumoconiosis (CWP). A lung disease with lesions, including deposits of carbon dust, along bronchioles. Bronchiolar widening due to loss of wall structure occurs. Chronic airway obstruction and bronchitis appear as disease progresses.

Coarctation of the Aorta. A congenital narrowing or constriction of the lumen of the aorta, which may occur anywhere along its length. Clinical manifestations vary according to location and extent of the constricture. Some patients are asymptomatic, but others experience headache, epistaxis, cold extremities, and claudication with exercise.

Coats' Disease. An exudative retinopathy occurring mostly in male children. It results in detached retina with severe vision loss.

Cocaine Abuse and Intoxication. ABUSE is evidenced by an individual who is intoxicated for a major portion of the day, may have episodes of cocaine overdose, and who is not able to either reduce or eliminate use. As a result of the pattern of use, interpersonal relationships and/or work productivity are adversely affected. INTOXICATION is manifested within one hour of use by symptoms that include euphoria, grandiosity, psychomotor agitation, pupillary dilatation, tachycardia, chills, and nausea and vomiting. Judgment and interpersonal relationships are adversely affected. Symptoms subside within twenty-four hours.

Coccidioidomycosis (Valley fever). A fungal lung infection. Mild, asymptomatic self-limited infection can occur. Symptomatic infections manifest fever, cough, chest pain, and malaise. Spontaneous improvement begins within two weeks and complete recovery is the rule.

Coccidiosis. An intestinal infection transmitted by the oral-anal route and resulting from the ingestion of undercooked infected pork or beef. Onset is usually acute and manifested by fever, headache, abdominal cramps, and diarrhea. Stools can be fatty and weight loss is common. Symptoms usually subside spontaneously but may persist for years and result in death.

Cockayne Syndrome. An inherited condition characterized by retinal degeneration, thick skin, photosensitivity, impaired hearing, short stature, and mental retardation.

Colitis. An inflammation of the colon caused by viruses, bacteria, or parasites. Clinical manifestations include fever, low abdominal cramps, and diarrhea, which can have blood in it. Many of the antibiotics may also cause mild to severe colitis.

Compulsion. Recurring impulses to perform a particular activity in a stereotyped way. The individual is unable to resist these impulses without experiencing extreme anxiety.

Compulsive Personality Disorder. A personality disorder characterized by long-standing patterns of behavior that adversely affect interpersonal relationshps and work productivity. Individuals with this disorder are task-oriented, overly concerned with details and order, have a need for things to be done their way, and do not express warm feelings freely. Although they tend to be "workaholics," their indecisiveness further limits their occupational effectiveness.

Conduct Disorder. A mental disorder that is usually diagnosed by the time the individual reaches adolescence and is more commonly found in males. The major characteristic is long-standing and recurring behaviors by which accepted legal and moral norms appropriate to the age group are defied. Typical behaviors include a pattern of lying, cheating, stealing, truancy, and running away from home. The individual usually functions below age level in school, is more limited in coping with frustration than is age appropriate, and evidences low self-esteem. There are four specific subtypes of the disorder based on the presence or absence of both social bonds and aggressive behavior.

Condyloma Acuminata. A viral disease resulting in the appearance of squamous papillomas on genitalia. Clinical manifestations include wartlike skin growths on the urethra, vulva, vagina, cervix, perineum, and anus. They may obstruct urination and defecation, may be subject to irritation and infection, and may become malignant.

Confabulation. The relating of information that has no basis in fact in order to compensate for lapses in memory. There is no conscious attempt to lie, as the individual believes the information is the truth.

Congestive Heart Failure. Circulatory congestion due to decreased myocardial contractility. Cardiac output is inadequate due to the inability of the heart to pump enough blood to meet the body's needs. Pulmonary vascular congestion and sodium and water retention result. Clinical manifestations include shortness of breath, dyspnea on exertion, paroxysmal nocturnal dyspnea, orthopnea, pitting edema of ankles and feet, distended neck veins, nocturia, liver congestion, and productive cough.

Conversion Disorder. A mental disorder usually characterized by an abrupt onset of physical symptoms following severe stress. The physical symptoms, which represent the conversion of a psychological conflict, enable the individual to both avoid the stressor and obtain support from significant others. The individual is unable to voluntarily control symptoms, the psychological conflict being at an unconscious level.

Coproporphyria. An inherited hepatic porphyria manifested by attacks of neuropsychiatric dysfunction and photosensitivity. Half of affected persons remain asymptomatic.

Cornelia de Lange Syndrome. An inherited malformation characterized by continuous eyebrows, thin down-turning upper lip, malformed hands and feet, hirsutism, short stature, and mental retardation.

Cor Pulmonale. A disease in which there exists hypertrophy of the right ventricle that is secondary to diffuse, extensive, and bilateral lung disease. Pulmonary atrial hypertension causes enlargement of the right ventricle. Clinical manifestations are those of right ventricular failure plus hypoxia.

Cretinism. Hypothyroidism dating from birth and resulting in developmental abnormalities such as hoarse cry, jaundice, constipation, somnolence, and feeding problems. There is belated growth and physical characteristics as follows: protruding tongue, broad flat nose, wide-set eyes, sparse hair, dry skin, and protruding abdomen with umbilical hernia. Mental development is also retarded.

Creutzfeldt-Jakob Disease. A fatal degenerative disease of the central nervous system. Onset occurs between ages forty to sixty and the course is rapidly progressive dementia with myoclonic seizures. The earliest symptoms include impairment of reasoning and judgment, memory disturbances, and bizarre behavior. Headaches, hallucinations, and confusion develop before the onst of clonic movements and convulsive episodes. Spasticity and rigidity also occur. Death occurs in three to twelve months from onset.

Crib Death. *See* Sudden Infant Death Syndrome.

Cribiform Hymen. A vaginal condition in which the hymen is thick and rigid with only multiple minute openings. Clinical manifestations include painful and blocked menses.

Cri-du-chat Syndrome. *See* Cat-Cry Syndrome.

Crigler-Najjar Syndrome. A congenital hyperbilirubinemia associated with brain damage and resembling kernicterus. Manifestations inlcude icterus, appearing shortly after birth, and neurological abnormalities.

Crohn's Disease (granulomatous colitis). A chronic inflammatory colitis. Clinical manifestations include fever, abdominal pain, diarrhea without urgency, and fatigability. Anorectal fistula and abscess formation are often the first presenting symptoms. Colonic malignancy is more common with these patients.

Croup. A viral infection resulting in acute epiglottitis, laryngitis, and laryngotracheobronchitis. Clinical manifestations include sudden onset of fever, sore throat, dysphagia, and severe respiratory distress with inspiratory stridor, hoarseness, brassy cough, and retractions.

Crouzon's Disease. An inherited craniofacial dysostosis characterized by acrocephaly, a beak-shaped nose, hypoplastic maxilla, short protruding lips, exophthalmos, and external strabismus.

Cushing's Syndrome. A condition resulting from, in most cases, bilateral adrenal hyperplasia secondary to hypersecretion of ACTH from the pituitary gland. The syndrome is characterized by truncal obesity, hypertension, fatigability, weakness, amenorrhea, hirsutism, purplish abdominal striae, edema, glucosuria, and osteoporosis. Deposition of adipose tissue in sites such as in the upper face "moon face" and in the interscapular area "buffalo hump" are characteristic.

Cyclothymic Disorder. A mental disorder characterized by a chronic disturbance in mood. There are both depressive and manic symptoms, but these are not as severe as those found in a major depression or a manic episode. Depressive and manic symptoms may be cyclical, mixed, or separated by an extended time period of relatively normal mood. There are no psychotic symptoms.

Cystic Fibrosis. An inherited disease (autosomal recessive) characterized by thick secretions from all mucous glands, pancreatic insufficiency, and an increase in the concentration of sodium and chloride in perspiration. There is a diffuse obstructive pulmonary process manifested by emphysema, atelectasis, and respiratory inflammation. Typical manifestations of this condition include persistent cough, failure to gain weight, excessive appetite, frequent bowel movements, growth retardation, pot belly, thick respiratory mucus, and anemia.

Cysticercosis. A pork tapeworm that has infected a human as its host. The worms develop in subcutaneous tissues, muscles, viscera, the eye, and the brain. Symptoms such as the following occur with heavy infestations: muscular pains, weakness, and fever. The symptoms of epilepsy, brain tumors, encephalitis, and psychiatric disorders may also appear.

Cystitis. An acute inflammation of the urinary bladder usually caused by a bacterium. One-half of the patients can be asymptomatic. Others manifest dysuria, frequency, urgency, and suprapubic pain. Urethritis is usually also present. The urine may be cloudy, malodorous, and bloody. The urethra is usually inflamed and tender.

Cytomegalic Inclusion Disease (CID) (salivary gland virus disease). A viral infection causing a broad spectrum of diseases. Categories of infections include congenital, neonatal, healthy children and adults, immunosuppressed patients, and organ-transplanted patients. Clinical manifestations vary and range from mononucleosislike symptoms to liver disease.

D

Deer-Fly Fever. *See* Tularemia.

Dejerine-Sottas Disease (hypertrophic polyneuropathy). An inherited slowly progressive nerve disease that starts in childhood. First clinical manifestations include pain and parathesia in the feet, followed by weakness and wasting of the distal limbs.

Delirium. A mental condition caused by organic factors such as metabolic disorders, systemic infections, head trauma, and substance intoxication or withdrawal. It is characterized by an altered level of consciousness, manifestations of which include disturbances in thinking, memory, and perception. There may also be disturbances in sleep patterns and psychomotor activity. The onset is usually rapid and symptoms tend to fluctuate.

Delirium Tremens. *See* Alcohol Withdrawal Delirium.

Delusion. A false and firmly held belief that is inconsistent with external reality. Despite contradictory evidence, the individual persists in maintaining the belief.

Delusional Syndrome, Organic. A mental condition caused by organic factors that include substances such as amphetamines and hallucinogens. It is characterized by the presence of delusions. The state of consciousness is not altered.

Dementia. A mental condition that is caused by organic factors. It is characterized by impairment of intellectual functioning as evidenced by losses in abstract thinking and judgment. Memory loss is prominent and may be accompanied by disorientation and changes in personality. Primary degenerative dementia, associated with Alzheimer's and Pick's diseases, is characterized by a gradual onset followed by slow but continuous deterioration. Multiinfarct dementia is associated with a rapid onset and is due to cerebrovascular disease.

Dementia associated with Alcoholism. *See* Alcoholism, Dementia associated with.

Dengue Fever. An endemic viral infection of tropical and subtropical areas of the world. The mosquito is the vector of transmission from human to human. Many patients are asymptomatic. Others may manifest fever with conjunctivitis, splitting headache, ocular pain, backache, and leg and joint pain. Skin rashes are also frequent.

Dependent Personality Disorder. A personality disorder characterized by long-standing patterns of behavior that adversely affect interpersonal relationships and may impair work productivity. It is manifested by a lack of self-confidence and an inability to be self-reliant or independent. Major decisions are passively permitted to be made by others and needs and desires are subordinated in order to maintain the dependent relationship.

Depersonalization. A feeling of unreality or strangeness about one's self. There is a sense of self-estrangement that may be accompanied by a feeling that one's body has an unreal quality. It is associated with a panic level of anxiety, severe stress, and some mental disorders.

Depersonalization Disorder. A mental disorder diagnosed only when episodes of depersonalization cause a disruption in interpersonal relationships or working abilities. The prominent characteristic is depersonalization, which may be accompanied by derealization. The onset of the disorder is usually during adolescence and may become chronic.

Depersonalization Neurosis. *See* Depersonalization Disorder.

Depressed Bipolar Disorder. *See* Bipolar Disorder, Depressed.

Depression, Major. An affective mental disorder characterized by the occurrence of a major depressive episode in an individual who has never had a manic episode. The major depressive episode is the distinct period of time in which symptoms of the disorder are present. Many individuals are symptom-free between episodes. The episodes are characterized by a persistent mood disturbance that leads to loss of interest in usual activities, thoughts of death or suicide, hopelessness, and helplessness. There may be accompanying sleep disturbances, changes in psychomotor activity and appetite, fatigue, and loss of interest in one's appearance. The individual may experience delusions or hallucinations.

Depressive Episode. *See* Depression, Major.

Depressive Neurosis. *See* Dysthymic Disorder.

Depressive Personality. *See* Dysthymic Disorder.

Derealization. A sensation of the environment having an unreal or strange quality that results in a loss of reality of the external world.

Dermatomyositis. A disease of unknown etiology affecting the striated muscle, skin, and connective tissues of the body. Clinical manifestations include painless weakness in the muscles such as in the hips and thighs, neck and shoulders, and quadriceps. A localized or diffuse erythema occurs. Weakness is progressive.

Dermatophytosis (Ringworm tinea). A chronic fungal infection of the skin, hair, and nails. The hand and foot infection (athlete's foot) present as fissuring between the toes, scaling, and vesicles. Scalp infection is characterized by areas of scaling and baldness. In the bearded area (tinea barbae) it presents as pustular folliculitis. In the nails, discoloration, thickening, and crumbling of nails occur.

Developmental Articulation Disorder. *See* Articulation Disorder, Developmental.

Developmental Language Disorder. *See* Language Disorder, Developmental.

Development Reading Disorder. *See* Reading Disorder, Developmental.

Devic's Disease. A variant of multiple sclerosis in which demyelination of the optic nerves and spinal cord occurs.

There may be a single episode with no further exacerbations.

Diabetes Insipidus. A condition resulting from lack of antidiuretic hormone (arginine vasopressin) usually caused by malfunction of the pituitary gland. The outstanding symptoms are polyuria and polydipsia. Dehydration, weight loss, anorexia, and hyperthermia can also occur.

Diabetes Mellitus. A metabolic disease of the Isles of Langerhans in the pancreas resulting in generalized hyperglycemia. The classical adult patient is overweight and presents with polydipsia, polyuria, increased appetite, weight loss, and sores that don't heal well.

DIC. *See* Coagulation, Disseminated Intravascular.

Diphtheria. An acute bacterial disease characterized by upper respiratory tract inflammation and by cardiac and neural effects resulting from the bacterial toxin. The incubation period is one to seven days, at which time the following manifestations occur: low fever, nausea and vomiting, inflammation and soreness of the throat with a typical grayish membrane formation over the throat. Hemorrhage occurs when attempts are made to remove the membrane. Overwhelming weakness and purpuric eruptions of the skin can occur. Myocarditis and peripheral neuritis can develop.

Disorganized Type, Schizophrenic Disorders. *See* Schizophrenic Disorders, Disorganized Type.

Disseminated Intravascular Coagulation. *See* Coagulation, Disseminated Intravascular.

Dissociative Disorders. Mental disorders characterized by responses to severe stress in which the individual dissociates or separates from awareness aspects of consciousness, identity, or motor behavior. The disorders include depersonalization disorder, multiple personality, psychogenic amnesia, and psychogenic fugue.

Diverticulitis. An inflammation of the diverticula or small herniations on the intestinal wall. Clinical manifestations include bowel irritability and irregularity, constipation, diarrhea, low abdominal cramps, low-grade fever and chills, and sudden massive hemorrhage.

Down's Syndrome (Mongolism). A congenital condition in which mental retardation of varying degrees and physical characteristics are present, such as small head with a sloping forehead, low-set oval ears, slightly slanted eyes, a medial epicanthal fold present, poorly developed bridge of the nose, enlarged tongue, shortened little fingers, and broad hands with a single transverse palmer crease. Stature is usually small and dwarflike. Mortality rate is high in the first year of life due to respiratory infections, cardiac anomalies, or leukemia.

Dracunculiasis. A guinea worm infection of connective and subcutaneous tissue. The parasite is transmitted in drinking water. Clinical manifestations include fever, generalized urticaria, periorbital edema, and wheezing. Subcutaneous blisters form around the adult worms causing pain and pruritis. Invasion of the joint tissue results in arthritis.

Dressler's Syndrome. A post-myocardial infarction syndrome. Onset is one to six weeks after a myocardial infarction and manifests as fever and chest pain, which radiates to the neck and shoulders and is relieved by leaning forward. Deep breathing exacerbates the pain. The syndrome is considered to be an autoimmune pericarditis, pleuritis, and pneumonitis. Salicylates and indomethacin bring prompt relief.

Dubin-Johnson Syndrome. An inherited condition in which there is a defect in biliary excretion. Clinically the liver may be enlarged and tender, and there may be vague constitutional or gastrointestinal symptoms.

Dubowitz Syndrome. A congenital malformation consisting of ptosis, shallow suborbital ridges, infantile eczema, short stature, and mental retardation.

Duchenne's Palsy. *See* Brachial Plexus Injury.

Dumping Syndrome. A syndrome, usually following peptic ulcer surgery, characterized by the following postprandial symptoms: palpitation, tachycardia, diaphoresis, abdominal pain, and vomiting. Symptoms occur approximately one-half hour after eating and are thought to be caused by a rapid emptying of hyperosmolar gastric juices into the small intestine.

Dwarfism. A condition of children in which there is an inadequate amount of growth hormone. Retardation of growth, epiphyseal development, and bone age results. Clinically there is increased truncal fat, puffy skin, long legs in relationship to the trunk, and retarded or absent sexual characteristics. The voice is high-pitched because of larynx maldevelopment.

Dyslexia. *See* Reading Disorder, Developmental.

Dysthymic Disorder (depressive neurosis). An affective mental disorder that usually starts in early adult life and tends to be chronic. It is characterized by periods of depressed mood or lack of interest in usual activities. Periods of time without depressive symptoms are usually limited to a few weeks. Symptoms are similar to, but are not as severe as those of a major depressive episode. There is no loss of contact with reality.

E

Eastern Equine Encephalitis. A viral infection transmitted from animals to man by the mosquito. Cases range from fatal central nervous system involvement to mild unreported illness. Clinically the patient may present with headache, fever, drowsiness, and convulsions. Nausea, vomiting, muscular pain, photophobia, nuchal rigidity, and tremors may also occur.

Eaton-Lambert Syndrome. A myasthenialike condition associated with carcinoma of the lung. There is pelvic, thigh, shoulder, and arm muscular weakness, aching, and stiffness. Ocular and bulbar muscles are usually unaffected. Tendon reflexes are depressed. The condition may precede the appearance of a malignant tumor by as much as two years.

Ebstein's Disease. A congenital cardiac anomaly consisting of downward displacement of an abnormal tricuspid valve into the right ventricle. Clinical manifestations include fatigue, cardiac dysrhythmias, cyanosis, cardiomegaly, and long systolic murmurs.

Echinococciasis. A worm infestation affecting mostly the liver and lungs and is transmitted from the intestinal tract of animals (principally dogs and sheep) to man. Clinically the symptoms depend upon the site, type, and size of the forming hydatid cysts. Cough, chest pain, and hemoptysis occur with lung lesions. Hepatic cysts cause jaundice, abdominal pain, and symptoms of acute cholecystitis.

Eclampsia. *See* Preeclampsia-Eclampsia.

Edward's Syndrome. A congenital abnormality manifested by neonatal hepatitis, scaphocephaly, small triangular mouth, micrognathia, blepharoptosis, low-set ears, mental retardation, hypertonicity, deafness, webbing of the neck, short stubby digits, overlapping of the index and third fingers, ventricular septal defect, and Meckel's diverticulum.

Ego-Dystonic Homosexuality. A psychosexual disorder of homosexuals who wish to develop heterosexual relationships, but who are aroused only by homosexual relationships. Homosexual arousal is persistent despite the individual's stated wishes and is extremely distressful.

Ehlers-Danlos Syndrome (cutis hyperelastica). An inherited abnormality of elastic tissue characterized by hyperelasticity and fragility of the skin, hyperextensibility of the joints, and a tendency to bleed easily.

Eisenmenger Syndrome. A congenital abnormality consisting of a combination of pulmonary hypertension and a communication between the aorta and lesser circulation resulting in elevation of pulmonary vascular resistance. Clinical manifestations include dyspnea, fatigue, feeding difficulties, failure to gain weight, and recurrent pneumonia.

Elliptocytosis. An inherited disease characterized by ovoid or elliptical-shaped red blood cells. Most patients manifest mild hemolysis with slightly lowered hemoglobin levels. Some patients, however, exhibit a substantially increased hemolysis resulting in enlarged spleens and anemia.

Ellis-van Creveld Syndrome (chondroectodermal dysplasia). An inherited condition characterized by hypoplasia of the teeth and nails, short distal limbs, polydactyly, small thorax, cardiac anomalies, and short statue.

Emphysema. A lung condition characterized by distention of the air spaces distal to the terminal bronchiole with alveolar septal damage. The condition has been associated with cigarette smoking, air pollution, and genetic factors. Clinical manifestations include dyspnea upon exertion, productive cough, and tachypnea with a prolonged expiration period through pursed lips and often accompanied by grunting. Neck veins may be extended and the intercostal spaces may retract with inspiration.

Encephalitis (sleeping sickness). An acute inflammatory process of the brain in which there is usually meningeal involvement. Cause is usually viral but may also be bacterial, fungal, parasitic, or syphilitic. Clinical manifestations include convulsions, confusion, stupor, coma, aphasia, hemiparesis, ataxia, involuntary movements, nystagmus, ocular palsies, and facial weakness associated with a high fever. Residual signs such as mental deterioration, amnesia, personality change, and hemiparesis may persist after resolution of the acute illness.

Encephalomyelitis. An acute encephalitis or myelitic process characterized by damage to the white matter of the brain or spinal cord. May follow measles, chickenpox, or rubella. The cause is thought to be a hypersensitivity reaction. Onset is usually abrupt presenting with headache, drowsiness, vomiting, and fever. Stiffness of the neck, flaccid paralysis, hemiplegia, loss of sphincter control, sensory loss, and coma may ensue.

Encephalotrigeminal Syndrome. Capillary or cavernous hemangiomas usually within cutaneous distribution of the trigeminal nerve. There occur a large number of abnormal blood vessels in the meninges and progressive destruction of the subjacent cortex. The first manifestation is usually a focal seizure on the side of the skin lesion followed by postictal paralysis. Frequent findings include paralysis, visual field defects, blindness in the eye on the side of the nevus, hemiparesis, and mental defects.

Enchondromatosis. *See* Ollier's Disease.

Encopresis, Functional. A childhood disorder in which a child past the age of four frequently defecates in inappropriate places. It is not related to any physical problem.

Endocardial Fibroelastosis. *See* Fibroelastosis, Endocardial.

Endocarditis. A microbial infection of the heart valves. Clinical manifestations include fever, cardiac murmurs, splenomegaly, anemia, hematuria, petechiae, and emboli. Weakness, night sweats, fatigability, anorexia, and arthralgia begin insidiously. Emboli may produce chest pain and vascular insufficiency may result in abdominal pain, sudden blindness, or pain in the extremities. Recent dental extraction, urethral instrumentation, respiratory infection, or surgery may precipitate an acute process.

Endometriosis. A benign condition characterized by the presence and proliferation of endometrial tissue in areas other than the endometrial cavity. It is reversible and regressive following ovarian inactivity and pregnancy. Clinical manifestations are variable and may include dysmenorrhea, pelvic pain, endometrial cysts, hemoperitoneum, abnormal uterine bleeding, dyspareunia, pain with defecation during menstruation, infertility, and obstruction and dysfunction of urinary and gastrointestinal tracts.

Enuresis, Functional. A childhood disorder in which a child past the age of four frequently urinates involuntarily during the day or night. It is not related to any physical problem.

Epidermolysis Bullosa. A congenital disorder characterized by the formation of blisters at the slightest sites of trauma. Blisters are slow to heal, become easily infected, and form scars. Infants may be born with large areas of erosion on their bodies. Mucous membranes may be involved and the nails may become thickened and clawlike.

Epilepsy. A condition characterized by recurrent convulsions, identical in type, that occur throughout the individual's entire lifetime. The cause is usually a cerebral lesion or other abnormality. Petit mal seizures come without warning and are characterized by a brief loss of consciousness. Blinks or jerks of the eyelids may be present. Grand mal seizures begin with a sudden loss of consciousness accompanied by an audible cry, a fall to the ground, tonic followed by clonic muscle contractions, and occasionally loss of sphincture control. A comatose state follows the motor activity and may last up to thirty minutes. Transient mental confusion, drowsiness, and headache occur as the patient regains consciousness.

Erb's Palsy. *See* Brachial Plexus Injury.

Erysipelas (St. Anthony's Fire). Streptococcal infection of skin and subcutaneous tissues. Commonly the face is affected. Onset is abrupt and manifestations include malaise, chills, fever, headache, and vomiting. Skin lesions begin as small itching areas of erythema that enlarge and spread for about three to six days. Vesicles and bullae may appear, rupture, and crust over. Recovery is usually present after a week, but the condition may become severe to fatal if bacteremia occurs.

Erysipeloid. A bacterial infection associated with traumatic dermal entrance into the body. The disease occurs mostly in people who work with dead animal products. Manifestations include a raised purplish-red zone surrounding the site of injury preceded by itching, burning, and pain in the area. Local swelling and joint stiffness and pain occur. The disease usually heals in about three days, but infective endocarditis may result if bacteremia occurs.

Erythroblastosis Fetalis. A hemolytic disease of newborns resulting from transplacental passage of maternal anti Rh antibody (when an Rh negative mother has been sensitized to an Rh positive infant). Clinical manifestation in the neonate include anemia, jaundice, pallor, and signs of cardiac decompensation and dissimated intravascular coagulopathy in severe cases.

Exhibitionism. A psychosexual disorder occurring in males that usually begins during the mid-twenties. It is characterized by sexual excitement being attained by exposing the genitals to a surprised stranger. This usually takes place in a public area and no additional sexual contact with the stranger is attempted.

F

Fabry Disease. An inherited x-linked enzyme ($\propto$-galacto-sidaso A) deficiency condition characterized by severe extremity pain, cutaneous angiokeratomas, corneal dystrophy, hypohidrosis, vascular thrombosis, and progressive fatal renal failure.

Factitious Disorders. Mental disorders in which psychological or physical symptoms are voluntarily controlled by the individual. Symptoms are deliberate and purposeful but have a compulsive quality. The only apparent goals are to be hospitalized and to assume a sick role. Psychological symptoms are diverse and become more severe when the individual knows that he or she is being watched. Symptoms include memory loss, hallucinations, and suicidal ideation. Additional symptoms are usually provided by the patient when questioned. Physical symptoms may similarly be total fabrications or may be the result of self-inflicted injury. The persistent presentation of diverse, physical symptomatology severe enough to obtain hospitalization is also known as Munchausen syndrome.

Failure to thrive. *See* Reactive Attachment Disorder of Infancy.

Fanconi Syndrome. A condition in which dwarfism and vitamin D-resistant rickets are present as well as aminoaciduria, renal glycosuria, hypophosphatemia, and hyperphosphaturia. Proteinuria, hyposthenuria, hypokalemia, and acidosis may also occur.

Farmer's Lung. A hypersensitivity pneumonitis caused by inhaling airborne material from moldy hay or vegetable matter. The acute form of this disease presents with malaise, chills, fever, nausea, cough, and dyspnea. Cyanosis, tachypnea, and tachycardia also are apparent. Chronically, there can be irreversible pulmonary fibrosis resulting in severe breathing problems.

Fascioliasis. A worm infestation of the bile duct contracted by ingestion of contaminated aquatic plants. Early symptoms include epigastric pain, fever, diarrhea, jaundice, urticaria, pruritis, and arthralgia, and are caused by migration of the larva to and within the liver. Obstruction of the bile ducts then occurs causing characteristic symptomatology.

Fasciolopsiasis. An upper intestinal infestation of flukes caused by ingesting aquatic plants that have been contaminated by pigs. Most patients are asymptomatic, but heavily infested persons exhibit abdominal pain, diarrhea, gastrointestinal hemorrhage, and intestinal obstruction. Asthenia with ascites and anasarca may appear at a later stage.

Feer's Disease. *See* Acrodynia.

Felty's Syndrome. The combination of rheumatoid arthritis, splenomegaly, and neutropenia. Vasculitis may occur and cause leg ulcers and peripheral neuropathy. Infection is a severe complication.

Fetishism. A psychosexual disorder characterized by sexual excitement being attained through use of inanimate objects. The disorder most commonly starts in adolescence and is usually chronic.

Fibrocystic Disease of the Breast. A diffuse and nodular fibrosis and formation of cysts also called "chronic cystic mastitis." It usually occurs in the later years of reproductive life. The condition is distinguishable from carcinoma because of the intermittent pain and resolution following each menstruation.

Fibroelastosis, Endocardial. A disease of unknown etiology characterized by a thickened endocardium with proliferation of elastic tissue. The left ventricle and the mitral and aortic valves are usually the most affected. Symptoms of congestive heart failure and stigmata of the congestive and restrictive forms of cardiomyopathy are manifested.

Fibrositis. A term used to denote a condition characterized by deep muscle and tendon aching and stiffness. Tender areas occur at characteristic points in the typical patient, who is elderly and depressed.

Fibrous Dysplasia. *See* Albright's Syndrome.

Fifth Disease (erythema infectiosum). A mild viral exanthematous condition with an incubation period of five to ten days. Manifestations include low-grade fever, erythema over the cheeks and later on the arms, legs, and trunk. The rash may come and go for weeks. Its reappearance can be brought on by heat, exercise, sunlight, or emotional stress.

Filariasis. A worm infestation of the lymphatics and subcutaneous tissues causing reactions from actue inflammation to chronic scarring. This species of worms can cause blindness, pruritic skin rash, and elephantiasis. Symptoms include lymphangitis with tenderness and swelling, and redness and swelling of the overlying skin, headache, nausea, vomiting, photophobia, and muscle pain. Abscesses may form about the lymph nodes and discharge to the surface.

Flight of ideas. Speech characterized by being rapid and almost continuous, with numerous sudden shifts in topics. Connections between topics may be through rhyming or a play on words.

Floppy-Valve Syndrome. *See* Systolic Click-Murmur Syndrome.

Folie à deux. *See* Paranoid Disorder.

Fort Bragg Fever. *See* Leptospirosis.

Fournier's Gangrene. An anaerobic cellulitis. Organisms spread along deep external fascial planes in the scrotum, peritoneum, and abdominal wall causing extensive loss of skin. There is a foul discharge present with marked pain, gas in the tissues, and systemic toxemia.

Froehlich's Syndrome. A hypothalamic disorder characterized by obesity, hypogonadotrophic hypogonadism in boys, diabetes insipidus, visual impairment, and mental retardation.

Fugue, Psychogenic. *See* Psychogenic Amnesia and Fugue.

Functional Encopresis. *See* Encopresis, Functional.

Functional Enuresis. *See* Enuresis, Functional.

G

Gambling, Pathological. A disorder that is characterized by an inability to control impulses to gamble over an extended period of time. The quality of family life is disturbed as financial losses from gambling may lead to arguments, borrowing money, and going heavily into debt without the resources to repay lenders. Work may also suffer with the individual who is absent during working hours in order to gamble.

Gamstrop's Disease. *See* Adynamia Episodica Hereditaria.

Gargoylism. *See* Hurler Syndrome.

Gas Gangrene. An aerobic bacterial disease that develops in traumatized tissue in which arterial circulation has been compromised such as wounds, constricting tourniquets or casts, compound fractures, surgical procedures, or foreign body penetrations. Symptoms include sudden severe pain, edema that feels hard to the touch, and cold, edematous distal limbs. There is brown watery drainage from the wound and a sweet characteristic odor followed by tiny gas bubbles. The infection may quickly become systemic and cause death.

Gastrinoma (Zollinger-Ellison Syndrome). A condition characterized by ulcers of the upper gastrointestinal tract, an increase in gastric acid, and islet cell tumors of the pancreas (gastrinomas). Clinical manifestations include symptoms that would be present in a patient who has gastric ulcers but of a more persistent, fulminating, and progressive type. Diarrhea may also be present due to large amounts of hydrochloric acid secreted from the stomach into the duodenum.

Gastritis. A condition of the stomach characterized by multiple bleeding areas of erosion. It can occur with no apparent cause but may be associated with aspirin ingestion and with severe stress secondary to burns, sepsis, trauma, surgery, shock, or renal failure. Patients present with hematemesis, epigastric pain, and nausea.

Gaucher's Disease. A genetic enzyme deficiency condition characterized by hepatosplenomegaly, hypersplenism, bleeding diathesis, bone pain, pathological fractures, and pulmonary problems. Severe neurological and/or pulmonary manifestation may cause an early death, but in many patients life span is not altered.

Gender Identity Disorder of Childhood. A psychosexual disorder characterized by strong, persistent desires to be or insistence that he or she actually is one of the other sex. The child's own anatomic structures are a source of distress. Activities more typical of the other sex are preferred. The onset of this uncommon disorder is before puberty.

German Measles. *See* Rubella.

Generalized Anxiety Disorder. *See* Anxiety Disorder, Generalized.

Giant Cell Arteritis. An inflammation of the arteries in the aged person. Cause is unknown. Symptoms include fever, sweats, malaise, fatigue, anorexia, and weight loss. Headache and aching pain and stiffness in the neck, shoulders, hips, and thighs often accompany this disease. Loss of vision can occur, forewarned by mild visual disturbances.

Giardiasis. A parasitic infestation of the duodenum and jejunum. The condition can be asymptomatic, but many patients exhibit nausea, flatulence, epigastric pain, abdominal cramps and distention, watery diarrhea, and weight loss. Transmission of the parasite is usually by infected water.

Gilbert's Syndrome. An inherited disease characterized by mild persistent unconjugated hyperbilirubinemia. It is usually not manifested until the patient is in his or her twenties when jaundice appears. The jaundice fluctuates and is worsened by fasting, surgery, fever, infection, or alcohol ingestion.

Gilchrist's Disease. *See* Blastomycosis.

Glanders. A bacterial infection that is transmitted to man by domestic animals. The incubation period is one to five days. Clinical manifestations include purulent discharge from the eyes, nose, and lips with ulcerating lesions, fever, rigors, myalgia, headache, pleuritic chest pain, photophobia, lacrimation, and diarrhea. The disease in an acute systemic form is often fatal.

Glaucoma. A condition of the eye in which high pressure in the aqueous humor is caused by an impediment to the outflow of aqueous fluid. The condition may go undetected for years and cause gradual damage to the optic nerve resulting in loss of peripheral vision and central vision acuity and eventual blindness. The patient may experience blurred vision, seeing "halos" around lights, and severe deep ocular pain with nausea and vomiting. The eyes may appear reddened with a hazy cornea and nonreactive pupil.

Glomerulonephritis, Acute (RGN). A kidney condition characterized by an abrupt onset of hematuria and proteinuria accompanied by azotemia and renal salt and water retention, leading to circulatory congestion, hypertension, and edema. Some of the causes include typhoid fever, sepsis, streptococcal and other bacterial infections, hepatitis, mumps, measles, lupus, Guillain-Barré syndrome, vaccinia, and malaria.

Glomerulonephritis, Chronic (CGN). A kidney syndrome characterized by chronic proteinuria, hematuria, and slowly progressive impairment of renal function leading to hypertension, granular kidneys, and end-stage renal failure. The causes are the same as in acute glomerulonephritis.

Glucagonoma. A hormone-secreting pancreatic tumor that causes a syndrome clinically characterized by a distinctive dermatosis called necrolytic migratory erythemia. Crusty, scaly macules and sometimes pustules are found on the face, lower abdomen, perineum, buttocks, and distal extremities. Exacerbations and remission of the rash occur and hyperpigmentation follows healing. Glossitis, stomatitis, weight loss, and normocytic anemia.

Gnathostomiasis. A parasitic tissue infestation. Clinical manifestations include migratory subcutaneous swellings and creeping eruptions. Migration into the central nervous system results in a lethal meningitis. Infestation is caused by eating diseased raw fish, duck, or chicken.

Goiter. An enlargement in the functioning thyroid mass and cellular activity brought about as a result of impairment of the thyroid gland capacity to secrete sufficient quantities of active hormones. Causes of the condition include iodine deficiency and cretinism. Clinical manifestations present as thyroid enlargement, mechanical displacement of the esophagus and trachea, and mediastinal obstruction.

Gonadal Dysgenesis. An inherited condition in which there is normal female genitalia but an absence of ovarian follicles resulting in sexual infantilism, primary amenorrhea, and hypoestrinism.

Gonorrhea. A bacterial infection of the epithelium. Direct contact of the urethra, anal canal, conjunctivas, pharynx, and endocervix transmit the bacteria. Local manifestations include endometritis, salpingitis, peritonitis, periurethral abscess and/or epididymitis. Systemically arthritis, dermatitis, endocarditis, meningitis, and hepatitis occur.

Goodpasture's Syndrome. A triad of findings of unknown etiology, which manifest as pulmonary hemorrhage, glomerulonephritis, and antibody to basement membrane antigens. Symptoms include cough, shortness of breath, hemoptysis, fever, and arthralgias. One of the most common clinical features is rapidly progressive renal failure.

Gout. A term describing a group of diseases that are manifested by high serum urate, recurrent attacks of characteristic arthritis, aggregated deposits of tophi (monosodium urate monohydrate) around the joints of the extremities, renal disease, and uric acid nephrolithiasis. Clinical symptoms include acutely painful arthritis, usually of the lower extremities and often involving the big toes, crystal urate (tophi) deposits appearing in the tissues, and urate crystal kidney stones.

Grandiosity. An exaggerated sense of one's own influence, knowledge, or worth.

Grave's Disease (Parry's or Basedow's disease). A triad of manifestations of unknown cause: hyperthyroidism with goiter, ophthalmopathy, and dermopathy; the three may not appear together. Clinically, the patient may present with goiter, fine tremor, emotional instability, excessive sweating, palpitations, hyperkinesis, loss of weight, weakness, eye manifestations, and localized pretibial myxedema.

Grippe. *See* Summer Grippe.

Guillain-Barré Syndrome (acute idiopathic polyneuritis). A syndrome of ascending motor paralysis of unknown cause. The principal clinical manifestations are a weakness that advances over a period of days and involves limb and trunk muscles, paresthesis, and facial diplegia. Prognosis is usually for complete recovery within a six- to eighteen-month period.

H

Hallerman-Streiff Syndrome. An inherited condition characterized by microphthalmia, cataracts, small pinched nose, thin skin over the nose, and short stature.

Hallervorden-Spatz Disease. An inherited condition usually manifesting in childhood or adolescence with abnormal muscle tone and rigid movements, dystonic posture, cerebellar ataxia and myoclonus, indistinct speech, and progressive intellectual impairment, with death usually occurring ten years after onset.

Hallucination. A sensory experience that occurs in the absence of external stimulation.

Hallucinogen Abuse. A substance-use disorder characterized by an individual who is not able to either decrease or eliminate usage, is intoxicated for major portions of the day dependent on the particular hallucinogen, and who may experience episodes of an affective or delusional disorder. Interpersonal relationships and work productivity are adversely affected by the pattern of use.

Hallucinogen Organic Mental Disorders. These include hallucinogen hallucinosis, a delusional disorder, and an affective disorder. Manifestations of HALLUCINOGEN HALLUCINOSIS include alterations in perception such as illusions, hallucinations, and depersonalization, which may be accompanied by poor judgment, depression, or heightened anxiety. Physical symptoms include incoordination, palpitations, pupillary dilation, tachycardia, and tremors. Symptoms usually appear in the first hour of use and most commonly last for about six hours, dependent on the specific hallucinogen. HALLUCINOGEN DELUSIONAL DISORDER is an organic delusional syndrome that lasts more than twenty-four hours after taking the hallucinogen. It can last varying amounts of time and can become a long-term psychotic episode. HALLUCINOGEN AFFECTIVE DISORDER is an organic affective syndrome that lasts more than twenty-four hours after taking the hallucinogen. It can last varying amounts of time and may be complicated by manic or major depressive episodes.

Hallucinosis, Organic. A mental syndrome that is caused by a specific organic factor such as LSD or persistent alcohol use. It is characterized by repeated hallucinatory experiences, the duration being dependent on the particular cause.

Hansen's Disease. *See* Leprosy.

Hartnup Disease. A genetic disorder that responds to massive doses of vitamin D. Clinical manifestations include mental retardation and cerebellar ataxia.

Hashimoto's Disease (lymphadenoid goiter). A chronic inflammation of the thyroid with possible autoimmune-factor involvement. Clinically, goiter is the main feature involving the entire gland. Hypothyroidism occurs as the condition progresses.

Heat Pyrexia (heat stroke, sunstroke, heat hyperpyrexia). A condition caused by hot weather and high humidity. Direct exposure to the sun is not a prerequisite. "Sweat fatigue" or a cessation of perspiration with hot skin occurs before the onset of symptoms. Symptoms include headache, vertigo, fatigue, abdominal cramping, confusion, hyperpnea, and often loss of consciousness. A rectal temperature of greater than 106 °F (41.1 °C) is not uncommon. Shock is common in fatal cases.

Hebephrenic Schizophrenia. *See* Schizophrenic Disorders, Disorganized Type.

Hemochromatosis. An iron storage disorder in which deposits of iron in parenchymal tissue results in damage and functional deficit in the involved organs. Excessive iron absorption or parenteral overload is often the cause. Clinically, hepatomegaly, pigmentation, spider angiomas, splenomegaly, arthropathy, ascites, cardiac dysrhythmias, congestive heart failure, loss of body hair, testicular atrophy, and jaundice are the outstanding manifestations.

Hemophilia. An inherited bleeding disorder in which there is a deficiency in blood clotting factor VIII (antihemophilic factor). Clinical manifestations vary depending upon the level of factor VIII activity. Signs include spontaneous recurrent bleeding associated with joint malformation, fever, anemia, and hyperbilirubinemia.

Hepatitis. Inflammation of the liver due to a viral infection. Two types of hepatitis have been identified: Hepatitis A, caused by virus A (also called infectious hepatitis, epidemic hepatitis, catarrhal jaundice, and short-incubation hepatitis); and Hepatitis B caused by virus B (also called serum hepatitis and homologous serum jaundice). Clinical manifestations include headache, fever, anorexia, nausea, vomiting, abdominal tenderness, pain over the liver, backache, myalgia, dark urine, and respiratory problems.

Hepatorenal Syndrome. Renal failure associated with advanced liver disease in the absence of other causes. Oliguria, urinary sediment, and low urinary sodium concentration occur. The mechanism of the renal failure is unknown and treatment is usually unsuccessful.

Herpes Simplex. A viral infection. Primary acute infection results in gingivostomatitis, rhinitis, keratoconjunctivitis, meningoencephalitis, and eczema. The transmission is by mucosal surface contact and the incubation period is two to twelve days. Sexual transmission is not uncommon.

Herpes Zoster (shingles). A viral infection characterized by segmental inflammation of the spinal and cranial nerves and by a painful localized skin eruption along the involved nerve routes. Chickenpox is also caused by the same virus.

Hiatal Hernia. A herniation of a portion of the stomach through the esophageal hiatus of the diaphragm. Symptoms mimic coronary insufficiency, cholelithiasis, peptic ulcer, and digestive disorders. Strangulation with acute prostration may occur.

Hippel-Lindau Syndrome. An inherited syndrome consisting of vascular malformation of the retina and cerebellum. Progressive loss of vision is caused by capillary angiomas. Progressive cerebellar ataxia, headache, and papilledema also occur. Manifestations usually first appear during adolescence.

Hirschsprung's Disease (aganglionic megacolon). A congenital condition characterized by absent bowel movements resulting in massive abdominal distention and chronic colonic obstruction resulting in malnutrition. The inability to defecate is caused by absence of neural intervention in a segment of the colon resulting in its inability to relax and pass stool.

Histoplasmosis. A fungal infection transmitted by inhalation of spores. Most infections are asymptomatic or mild. Signs and symptoms include cough, fever, and malaise. The disease may become chronic with pulmonary necrosis and calcification mimicking tuberculosis. Chronic infection causes weight loss, night sweats, and an increasingly productive cough. Emphysema, cor pulmonale, or pneumonia can be complicating factors that may cause death.

Histrionic Personality Disorder. A personality disorder characterized by long-term patterns of behavior in which individuals are consistently overly dramatic, prone to emotional outbursts, draw attention to themselves, and are emotionally labile. Interpersonal relationships are limited by their being self-centered, self-indulgent, shallow, and dependent.

Hodgkin's Disease. A malignant disease of lymphoreticular system. Clinical manifestations include painless enlargement of the lymph nodes, remittent fever, night sweats, weight loss, persistent dry cough, and malaise. Slow progression of the disease leads to tumor invasion of pulmonary parenchyma, blood vessels, spleen, liver, and other viscera.

Homocystinuria. A congenital abnormality characterized by an increase in the concentration of the sulfur-containing amino acid, homocystine, in blood and urine. Mental retardation, osteoporosis, thrombotic vascular disease, and central nervous system dysfunction can result.

Homosexuality, Ego-Dystonic. *See* Ego-Dystonic Homosexuality.

Horner Syndrome. A lesion of the cervical sympathetic nerve fibers characterized by ptosis, meiosis, and absence of sweating on the affected side of the face.

Huntington's Chorea. A genetic disorder (mendelian dominant trait) eventuating in progressive dementia, bizarre involuntary movements (chorea), and unusual postures. Manifestations generally start to appear in the third or fourth decade and progressively worsen. The patient presents with respiratory irregularities, grimacing, faulty speech, bizarre and irregular limb movements, and rigidity. The disease terminates in death after many years.

Hurler Syndrome (gargoylism). An inherited metabolic disturbance. Clinical features include a malformed skull, profuse nasal discharge, short neck, enlarged tongue, kyphosis, enlarged heart, absence of sexual maturation, characteristic "clawing" fingers, limited joint extensibility, corneal opacities, and mental retardation.

Hyaline Membrane Disease. *See* Respiratory Distress Syndrome.

Hydatidiform Mole. A degenerative transformation of gestational trophoblastic tissue that can become malignant. Clinical characteristics include hydropic villi, bleeding during the first trimester, disproportionate uterine growth, hypertension, proteinuria, low abdominal pain, excessive nausea and vomiting, visual disturbances, edema, excessive weight gain, and passage of characteristic clear grapelike vesicles.

Hydrocephalus. A condition in which enlargement of the cerebral ventricular system occurs as a result of an imbalance between production and absorption of cerebral spinal fluid. Clinical manifestations depend upon time of onset. If in infancy, suture separation, dilated scalp vein, cranial enlargement, high-pitched cry, and downward deviated eyes occur. If late onset, spasticity, ataxia, urinary incontinence, and progressive decline in mental activity occur.

Hymenolepiasis. A dwarf tapeworm infestation. Clinical manifestations include gastrointestinal and allergic symptoms.

Hyperactive Child Syndrome. *See* Attention Deficit Disorder.

Hyperparathyroidism. An increased secretion of parathyroid hormone from the gland leading to hypercalcemia and hypophosphatemia. Clinical manifestations include recurrent nephrolithiasis, peptic ulcer disease, mental changes and excessive bone resorption. Muscle weakness, fatigability, and muscle atrophy occur as well as calcification of the cornea of the eye. Most cases are the result of benign neoplasm or hyperplasia.

Hypertension. A condition in which the systolic and/or diastolic blood pressure is elevated because of abnormally small vessels in the arterial system. Primary or essential hypertension occurs when other causes of hypertension are absent in the presence of a diastolic pressure of 90 mm Hg. or higher. Secondary hypertension follows other pathology. Clinical manifestations include elevated blood pressure on three different occasions, vascular changes in the capillaries of the eye, headache, muscle cramps, and palpitation.

Hyperthyroidism. A condition caused by overproduction of the thyroid hormones and resulting in toxic goiter. Clinical manifestations include adenomas, nervousness, hyperexcitability, irritability, apprehension, tachycardia, low heat tolerance, flushed skin, profuse perspiration, fine hand tremors, exophthalmos, increased appetite with progressive weight loss, weakness, and amenorrhea.

Hypochondriasis (hypochondriacal neurosis). A mental disorder characterized by a preoccupation with one's state of health, accompanied by various and persistent symptoms that occur in the absence of any demonstrable physical condition. The course of the disorder is usually chronic as the individual is unable to accept any reassurances that a disease is not present and may eventually assume an invalid life style.

Hypomania. A clinical syndrome in which symptoms resemble but are not as severe as those of a manic episode (*see* Bipolar Disorder, Manic).

Hypoparathyroidism. A condition resulting from diminution or absence of the parathyroid hormones. Blood calcium falls and blood phosphate elevates. Clinical manifestations include tetany, facial muscle spasms (Chvostek's sign), carpopedal spasm (Trousseau's sign), laryngeal spasm, and renal colic.

Hypospadias. A congenital abnormality of the penis in which the urethral orifice is located on the ventral surface.

Hysterical Neurosis, Conversion Type. *See* Conversion Disorder.

Hysterical Personality. *See* Histrionic Personality Disorder.

I

Ideas of reference. Unwarranted ideas that particular incidents, objects, or other people have a special significance for the individual. Ideas of reference are not believed as strongly as are delusions.

Identity Disorder. A mental disorder that is characterized by persistent uncertainties and lack of trust in one's self and is manifested by impaired abilities to make decisions involving major issues such as career choice, friendships, long-term goals, religious values, and sexual orientation. The disorder usually begins during late adolescence.

Idiopathic Hypertrophic Subaortic Stenosis (IHSS) or asymmetric septal hypertrophy (ASH). A familial cardiac abnormality characterized by marked hypertrophy of the left ventricle, most strikingly in the septal area causing obstruction to outflow and a decrease in velocity of contraction. Clinical manifestations include dyspnea, angina, syncope, and left ventricular failure.

Illusion. A misinterpretation of an actual external sensory stimulus.

Impetigo Contagiosa. A streptococcal pyoderma that is easily spread and highly contagious. Clinical features include superficial crusted or blisterlike lesions.

Infantile Autism. An uncommon disorder that is manifested in infancy. There is a lack of responsiveness and a lack of formation of close attachments to significant others. As the infant grows, there is a lack of development of normal communication patterns, both verbal and nonverbal. Ritualistic behavior, fascination with motion, and extraordinary resistance to minor changes in routine are also found. The disorder is chronic.

Infantile Paralysis. *See* Poliomyelitis.

Infantile Spinal Muscular Atrophy (Werdnig-Hoffman disease). An inherited disorder characterized by atrophy of anterior horn cells in the spinal cord, motor nuclei in the brain stem, motor nerve roots, and muscles. Manifestations include weakness and hypotonia of the limbs, froglike lying position, absent tendon reflexes, and intercostal muscle weakness resulting in respiratory failure and death.

Infundibular Stenosis. A congenital cardiac abnormality characterized by failure of involution of the bulbus cordis resulting in obstruction in the outflow tract of the right ventricle. Clinical manifestations mimic those of acyanotic tetralogy of Fallot.

Intussusception. A condition in which there is an invagination of a portion of the intestine into a distal adjacent part. It usually occurs during the ages three to twenty-four months. Clinical manifestations include sudden severe paroxysmal pain, straining efforts, weakness, high fever, vomiting, "currant-jelly" stools, abdominal mass upon palpitation, and abdominal distention and tenderness.

Involutional Melancholia. *See* Depression, Major.

J

Jakob-Creutzfeldt Disease. A fatal degenerative disease of the central nervous system transmitted by contact with blood or cerebrospinal fluid of an infected patient. Clinical manifestations first appear as mental changes such as memory loss, bizarre behavior, hallucinations, confusion, and visual distortions. Convulsions, ataxia, disarthria, muscular atrophy, spasticity, and rigidity appear later. The disease progresses rapidly to death.

Jeune Syndrome (asphyxiating thoracic dystrophy). A congenital condition characterized by very short ribs, polydactyly, and cleftlike lesions in the acetabulum and metaphyses of the long bones. The thorax is narrow and immobile and breathing is limited.

Juvenile Retinoschisis. An inherited degenerative eye disease characterized by a splitting of the retina into two layers. Vision is slowly and progressively lost.

K

Kala Azar. A leishmaniasis infestation transmitted from animals to man by the bite of a sandfly. The incubation period is ten days to one year. Clinical manifestations include a primary "chancre" that heals with scarring, fever that is characterized by two daily spikes, progressive weakness, weight loss, tachycardia, hyperpigmentation, and edema due to portal hypertension. Mortality in untreated patients is high.

Kaposi's Sarcoma. A skin malignancy. Lesions usually begin on the feet, ankles, hands, and arms, and progress proximally. Extracutaneous lesions are found in the GI and respiratory tracts, where they can result in bleeding.

Kearn's Syndrome. An inherited condition characterized by chronic progressive external ophthalmoplegia, pigmentary degeneration of the retina, cardiomyopathy, weakness of facial, laryngeal and trunk muscles, deafness, and small stature.

Kinky Hair Syndrome. *See* Menke's Syndrome.

Kleptomania. A disorder of impulse control in which the individual is unable to resist impulses to steal. The items stolen are not needed by the individual, who is able to pay for them. Prior to the theft, the individual has a sensation of heightened tension that is released and may be accompanied by a sense of pleasure as the actual theft takes place.

Klinefelter Syndrome. A genetic abnormality characterized by mental retardation, nervousness, immature behavior, small testes, delayed puberty, infertility, and a tall, slim, and underweight stature.

Korsakoff's Disease. *See* Alcohol Amnestic Disorder.

Krabbe's Disease. An inherited condition consisting of cerebroside lipidosis or globoid leukodystrophy. Clinical manifestations include rigidity, hyperreflexia, swallowing difficulties, and motor and intellectual development problems.

Krukenberg's Tumor. A primary mesenchymal malignant tumor of the ovary that is usually a result of metastasis from a primary stomach carcinoma.

Kwashiorkor. A protein-energy undernutritional disease in which calories are adequate but protein is deficient. Manifestations include growth failure and mental retardation in children, edema, fatty liver, preservation of adipose tissue, and blanched or reddish hair.

L

Landouzy-Dejerine Dystrophy. A faciocapulohumeral muscular dystrophy differing from other dystrophies because of the presence of facial muscle weakness involving all the facial muscles. Asymmetric movements of the mouth are particularly characteristic. Weakness of the muscles of the pectoral girdle with winging of the scapulae is also present. Characteristically the patient cannot raise the entire arm, but strength in the forearm and hand is maintained.

Language Disorder, Developmental. Includes expressive and receptive disorders. An EXPRESSIVE DISORDER is characterized by a child's inability to develop fully and express language at his or her age level despite the ability to understand. A RECEPTIVE DISORDER is characterized by lack of development of both comprehension and verbal expression despite normal nonverbal I.Q.

Latent Schizophrenia. *See* Schizotypal Personality Disorder.

Laurence-Moon-Biedl Syndrome. An inherited condition characterized by obesity, polydactyly, retinal pigmentation, mental deficiency, and short stature.

Legionnaires' Disease. An acute bacterial respiratory infection. Incubation period is two to ten days. Clinical manifestations include fever, myalgia, headache, pneumonia with a progressively productive cough, dyspnea, and pleuritic chest pain. GI symptoms, including nausea, vomiting, diarrhea, and cramps, may also be present. The major complication is respiratory failure and when this is present, mortality is high.

Leigh's Syndrome. An inherited pyruvic acid carboxylase defect resulting in progressive encephalopathy. Clinical manifestations are variable and may include progressive mental retardation, failure to thrive, seizures, vomiting, and respiratory difficulty.

Leishmaniasis. A protozoan infestation transmitted to man by the bite of a sandfly. The infestation may be either visceral with recurrent fever, splenomegaly, pancytopenia, weight loss and high mortality; or cutaneous with chronic skin ulcers, destructive mucotaneous lesions, and a leprosy-like infection.

Leopard Syndrome. *See* Moynalian's Syndrome.

Leprechaunism (Donohue syndrome). An inherited condition characterized by extreme growth deficiency with large hands and feet, enlarged phallus, hirsutism, and full lips.

Leprosy (Hansen's disease). A chronic granulomatous bacterial infection that affects superficial tissues, peripheral nerves and nasal mucosa. Clinical manifestations include hypo- or hyperpigmented macules or plaques on the skin, or anesthetic or paresthetic skin patches in the early stages. Enlarged peripheral nerves, neuritic pain, muscular atrophy, hand and foot contractures, loss of phalanges, and blindness occur later. Septal perforation and nasal collapse and lymphadenopathy are not uncommon.

Leptomeningitis. *See* Meningitis, Bacterial.

Leptospirosis (Fort Bragg fever). A disease of infestation by leptospiras, which are transmitted to man from water contaminated by animal urine. Clinically the disease is biphasic. During the first phase there is an abrupt onset of headache, muscle aching, myalgia, high fever, and chills. Nausea and vomiting, diarrhea, and coughing and chest pain can also occur. In the second phase, after an asymptomatic period of one to three days, fever, meningismus, optic neuritis, encephalitis, myelitis, and peripheral neuritis may occur.

Lesch-Nyhan Disease. An inherited enzymatic disorder characterized by mental retardation, choreoathetoid movements, scissoring position of the legs, self-mutilation, and overproduction of uric acid.

Leukemia. A disease characterized by neoplastic growth of one of the blood-forming cells. The leukemias are classified according to the involved cell type. Possible contributing factors to this disease include large doses of radiation, chemical agents, viruses, and hereditary factors. Clinical manifestations are related to replacement of normal cells of the blood by leukemic cells and include high fever, prostration, bleeding, recurrent local infections, bone and joint pain, muscle wasting, contractures, weight loss, and extreme pallor.

Leukodystrophy. An inherited (autosomal recessive) degenerative diffuse cerebral sclerosis. Clinical manifestations are progressive dementia, weak and unsteady gait, spasticity, and hypotonia.

Lightwood Syndrome. *See* Albright's Syndrome.

Lignac Syndrome (cystinosis). Fanconi syndrome with added presence of cystine crystals in the body tissues.

Lindau's Disease. A familial kidney disorder characterized by the presence of cysts or adenomas of the kidney, cysts of the pancreas, and hemangiomas of the retina, cerebellum, brain stem, or spinal cord.

Listeriosis. A bacterial infection mostly affecting infants under one month of age. Transplacental perinatal infection can result in stillborn or premature birth. Clinical manifestations include meningitis, cardiorespiratory distress, dark red skin papules on lower extremities, and hepatosplenomegaly.

Little's Disease. A form of cerebral palsy associated with prematurity or difficult parturition. Quadriplegia, mental retardation, spastic paraplegia, upper motor disturbances, and diminished head size are the types of manifestations that are present.

Loiasis. A form of filariasis that is transmitted by deer flies. Calabar swellings of the subcutaneous tissue are hallmarks of the disease. Worms in the conjunctivae can result in pain and lacrimation. Endomyocardial fibrosis has been reported as being associated with this infestation.

Lockjaw. *See* Tetanus.

Loosening of associations. Speech based on thinking in which ideas expressed shift from topic to topic without any connection or logical association.

Lupus Erythematosus. A disease of unknown cause predominantly occurring in women. The hallmark of the disease is the presence of many antibodies to nuclear antigens (ANA) forming immune-complexes that explain the multitude of problems. Clinical manifestations include arthritis and arthralgias, discoid lupus, renal involvement, cardiopulmonary abnormalities, neurological disorders, and enlarged lymph nodes.

M

Major Depression. *See* Depression, Major.

Malaria. A protozoan disease transmitted to man by the bite of the *Anopheles* mosquito. The incubation period is from ten to fourteen days. General manifestations include the malarial paroxysm (begins with chills, followed by very high fever, and ends with profuse diaphoresis), splenomegaly, mental confusion, edema, postural hypotension, severe anemia, headache, and myalgia.

Mallory-Weiss Syndrome. Lacerations in the region of the esophagogastric junction often following retching or nonbloody vomiting. The result can be profuse hemorrhage manifested by hematemesis.

Manic Bipolar Disorder. *See* Bipolar Disorder, Manic.

Manic Depressive Illness. *See* Bipolar Disorder.

Manic Episodes. *See* Bipolar Disorder, Manic.

Marfan Syndrome (arachnodactyly). An inherited generalized disease of the supporting tissues of the ocular, cardiovascular, and skeletal systems. Clinically the patient manifests bilateral subluxation of the lens (ectopia lentis), uveitis, glaucoma, cataracts, dissecting aneurysm of the ascending aorta, severe mitral valve regurgitation, aortic valve abnormalities, increased length of the tubular bones, weakness of the tendons, recurrent dislocations, kyphoscoliosis, and inguinal hernias.

Masochism, Sexual. *See* Sexual Masochism.

McArdle Syndrome. An enzymatic disorder of glycogen metabolism characterized by muscle weakness and pain following exercise.

McCune-Albright Syndrome. A sporatic condition of unknown cause characterized by the triad of polyostotic fibrous dysplasia, café-au-lait spots, and isosexual percocity. Cushing's syndrome, gigantism, or acromegaly may also occur.

Measles. *See* Rubeola.

Meckel-Gruber Syndrome. An inherited condition characterized by encephalocele, polydactyly, polycystic kidneys, mental retardation, and short stature.

Meckel's Diverticulum. An outpouching of the ileum close to the ileocecal valve. Clinical manifestations include bleeding, anemia, and abdominal pain.

Mediterranean Fever (paroxysmal polyserositis). An inherited condition of unknown etiology. A variable syndrome that usually has its onset between the ages of five to fifteen. The characteristic attacks consist of chills, followed by fever and ending with diaphoresis. Abdominal pain, acute pleuritic pain, joint pain, and erythematous swellings of the skin may also be present.

Megaloblastic Anemia. A blood disorder of erythroid maturation. Megaloblastic red blood cells tend to be large and vulnerable to destruction. The most common causes are vitamin B_{12} and folic acid deficiencies. Clinical features include weakness, vertigo, tinnitus, palpitations, angina symptoms of congestive heart failure, pallor, numbness, paresthesis, poor finger coordination, decreased reflexes, sore tongue, weight loss, and GI disturbances.

Melioidosis. A bacterial glanderslike infection transmitted to man from the soil by inhalation, ingestion, and contamination of skin abrasions. Clinical manifestations include fever, malaise, lymphadenitis, headache, myalgia, pleuritic chest pain, cough, pneumonia, arthritis, meningitis, and enlarged liver and spleen.

Melkersson Syndrome. A condition of unknown cause in which attacks of seventh (facial) cranial nerve weakness occur in conjunction with edema of the lips.

Menetrier's Disease. A type of gastric mucosal hyperplasia of unknown cause. It is characterized by extreme tortuous enlargement of the gastric mucosal folds. The patient complains of epigastric pain, anorexia, nausea, vomiting, weight loss, and diarrhea.

Meniere's Syndrome. A degeneration of the ear's vestibular and cochlear hair cells characterized by recurrent vertigo, tinnitis, and deafness. Usually the deafness is progressive and when it is total, the vertigo ceases.

Meningitis, Bacterial (leptomeningitis). An inflammation of the piarachnoid and contamination of cerebrospinal fluid thus affecting the ventricles of the brain and spine. Symptomatology includes fever, headache, seizures, stiff neck and back, confusion, and delirium. Petechial and purpuric skin eruptions and ecchymosis of the lower extremities are characteristic.

Meningomyelocele. *See* Spina Bifida.

Menke's Syndrome (kinky hair syndrome). An inherited disorder of copper metabolism. Cerebral degeneration and arterial changes cause death in infancy. Clinical manifestations include failure to gain weight, hypothermia, sparse and brittle scalp hair, seborrheic dermatitis, seizures, and severe developmental retardation.

Mental Disorder. A psychological or behavioral pattern occurring in an individual who is unable to adequately function in major aspects of daily living such as work or interpersonal relationships. The impaired functioning causes distress to the individual and may be evidenced by behavioral, biological, or psychological symptoms.

Mental Retardation. A disorder in which intellectual functioning is significantly below average. It is characterized by the individual's impaired ability to function as compared to others of similar age and culture. The majority (80 percent) are mildly retarded with I.Q. levels of 50–70 and are educable. It may be diagnosed in some shortly after birth, the onset always being before age eighteen.

Meralgia Paresthetica Syndrome. A compression of the lateral cutaneous nerve of the thigh that may develop in obese pregnant women. Clinical features include paresthesias and loss of sensation over the anterolateral aspect of the thigh, which are initiated by walking and prolonged standing.

Middle Lobe Syndrome. A condition consisting of pneumonitis, bronchial obstruction, and atelectasis.

Migraine. A periodic, hemicranial throbbing headache. Before the onset of the headache, nausea and vomiting, visual disturbances, slight speech abnormalities, and hemiparesis can occur. Vasodilatation and excessive pulsation of external carotid artery branches are thought to be caused by a release of amines bringing on the migraine.

Mikulicz's Disease. A painless enlargement of the salivary gland simulating a neoplasm. It usually occurs in adult women but may also occur in childhood.

Milk Sickness. A condition caused by ingestion of milk or meat from an animal that has been poisoned by eating certain toxic goldenrods or snakeroot. Clinical symptoms include nausea, vomiting, constipation, jaundice, anuria, dark red tongue, red, flushed lips and cheeks, abdominal pain, and muscular weakness. Convulsions may lead to death.

Minimal Brain Damage. *See* Attention Deficit Disorder.

Mixed Bipolar Disorder. *See* Bipolar Disorder, Mixed.

Moebius Syndrome. A congenital absence or maldevelopment of cranial nerves. Clinical manifestation include ptosis, complete ophthalmoplegia, inability to close the eyes, swallowing and chewing difficulties, and an expressionless, immobile face.

Mondor's Disease. Thrombosis of the thoracoepigastric veins and sclerosing subcutaneous phlebitis. This condition occurs after trauma. There is no known cause. Symptomatology includes tender, long cordlike structures in the outer half of the breast. They usually disappear within a year.

Mongolism. *See* Down's Syndrome.

Moniliasis. *See* Candidiasis.

Mononucleosis. A lymphotropic herpes viral infection. Incubation period is thirty to fifty days. Frank clinical symptoms include fever, sore throat, lymph node enlargement, splenomegaly, fatigue, and malaise.

Mood. A prolonged emotional state, more enduring and persuasive than affect. Usual descriptions may include anxious, angry, depressed, happy, or irritable.

Moynahan's Syndrome (Leopard syndrome). A genetic (autosomal dominant) disorder characterized by multiple small, circumscribed hypermelanotic macules. EKG abnormalities, occular hypersteloriom, pulmonary stenosis, genitalia abnormalities, deafness, and growth retardation are also manifestations.

Mucormycosis. An acute fungal infection producing a typical clinical picture of fever, dull sinus pain, nasal congestion or discharge, double vision, and obtundation with pneumonia.

Mucosal Neuroma Syndrome. Multiple mucosal neuromas associated with thyroid carcinoma. Neurofibromas occur on the tongue, mouth, lips, conjunctiva and intestines. Café-au-lait patches may be present. Patients may be tall with scoliosis, pectus excavatum, pes cavus, muscular hypotonia, and arachnodactyly. Pheochromocytoma and hyperthyroidism are also present.

Multi-Infarct Dementia. *See* Dementia.

Multiple Myeloma. A disseminated malignancy of plasma cells associated with bone destruction, bone marrow failure, hypercalcemia, renal failure, and recurrent infections. The hallmark is bone pain from pathological fractures.

Multiple Personality. A dissociative disorder in which two or more complete personalities exist within an individual. The personalities are usually very different from each other, and each one may become dominant at a particular time. The disorder is relatively rare.

Multiple Sclerosis. A disease of demyelination of certain portions of the nervous system, spinal cord, optic nerves, and brain. Clinical episodes remit and recur over a period of twenty to thirty years. Clinical features include impaired vision, nystagmus, dysarthria, tremor, ataxia, limb weakness, bladder dysfunction, and paraplegia.

Mumps. An acute viral infection. The route of communicability is respiratory, and the incubation period is fifteen to twenty-one days. The hallmark feature of mumps is parotitis accompanied by fever, malaise, headache, and anorexia. Complications that can occur include epididymoorchitis resulting in sterility, pancreatitis, meningitis, oophoritis, and myocarditis.

Munchausen Syndrome. *See* Factitious Disorders.

Myasthenia Gravis. A disease of muscular weakness resulting from a functional abnormality at the neuromuscular junctions. Clinical characteristics include weakness of laryngeal and pharyngeal muscles with choking and aspiration of food, limb muscle weakness, typical fatigability with relief of weakness after rest, drooping eyelids, and abnormal speech. The muscular weakness usually responds to rest and anticholinesterase drugs.

Myocardial Infarction. An area of myocardial tissue destruction due to compromised blood flow through the coronary arteries caused by a thrombus or atherosclerosis. Clinical manifestations of the acute phase include steady constrictive chest pain, arrhythmias, profuse perspiration, moist clammy skin, dyspnea, weakness, fainting, nausea and vomiting, anxiety, hypotension, and shock.

N

Nail-Patella Syndrome. A genetic (autosomal dominant) disorder characterized by dystrophic nails, absence of one or both patellae, ilicic horns, and progressive renal failure.

Narcissistic Personality Disorder. A personality disorder characterized by long-standing patterns of behavior in which the individual displays an overestimation of his or her abilities and an inflated self-importance, and demands attention and admiration. Relationships with others are characterized by a lack of empathy, exploitation, and the expectation of favors without any thoughts of reciprocating.

Narcolepsy. A syndrome characterized by recurring attacks of inability to remain awake. Overpowering sleep comes on suddenly while the person is engaged in activity. The sleep is shallow and the patient easily aroused.

Neologisms. New words invented by an individual that may have subjective meanings that are not comprehended by others. Common words may also be distorted and new meanings given to them.

Nephritis. A term describing various diseases involving inflammation of the kidney glomeruli. The results lead to hypertension, pulmonary vascular congestion, and facial and peripheral edema.

Nephroblastoma. *See* Wilm's Tumor.

Nephrotic Syndrome. A disorder of increased permeability of the glomerular basement membrane to protein. Characteristics include edema, hypoproteinemia, hyperlipidemia, and excessive proteinuria.

Neurotic Disorders. Mental disorders characterized by symptoms that either express anxiety or are the result of behaviors adopted to cope with anxiety. There is no gross distortion of external reality. Symptoms are both distressful and unacceptable to the individual and tend to be chronic. (As the American Psychiatric Association has recategorized the neurotic disorders, they are described in this text under those new headings and are cross-referenced to previously used titles.)

Noonan Syndrome. A genetic disorder characterized by features of narrow maxilla, small mandible, triangular-shaped mouth, epicanthic eye folds, ptosis, downward slant of the eyes, prominent ears, webbing of the neck, multiple pigmented nevi, dystrophic nails, and short stature. Cardiac abnormalities, mental retardation, infertility, and hydronephrosis may also be present.

Norrie's Disease. An inherited condition characterized by blindness, mental retardation, deafness, and degeneration of the central nervous system.

O

Obsession. Repetitive thoughts that invade consciousness and are not wanted. They are repugnant to the individual who attempts to ignore or suppress them.

Obsessive Compulsive Disorder (obsessive compulsive neurosis). An anxiety disorder characterized by the presence of either obsessions or compulsions. These are extremely disturbing to the individual, severely limiting activities of daily living and interpersonal relationships. The disorder is uncommon, most frequently starts in early adulthood, and tends to be chronic.

O'Hara's Disease. *See* Tularemia.

Ollier's Disease (enchondromatosis). A bone disorder in which hypertrophic cartilage is not resorbed and ossified normally. Clinical characteristics usually appear in childhood and include unilateral deformities and retardation in bone growth, usually in the long bones and pelvis.

Onchocerciasis (River blindness). A cutaneous filariasis characterized by subcutaneous nodules enclosing adult worms, pruritis, keratitis, and iridocyclitis. Blindness may occur as well as chronic thickening, lichenification, and depigmentation of the skin.

Opioid Abuse and Dependence. ABUSE is a substance-use disorder characterized by an inability to decrease or eliminate usage, intoxication during large portions of the day, and almost daily use. Work productivity and interpersonal relationships are adversely affected as a direct result of the pattern of use. DEPENDENCE is characterized by either the development of withdrawal symptoms with a decrease or elimination of usage or by having to take increasingly larger amounts of opioids in order to maintain the needed effects.

Opioid Organic Mental Disorders. These include intoxication and withdrawal. Signs of opioid INTOXICATION include euphoria, pupillary constriction, psychomotor retardation, poor judgment, slurred speech, memory loss, and decreased attention span. Effects usually last four to six hours. Signs of opioid WITHDRAWAL, following a decrease or elimination after long-standing opioid use, include diarrhea, fever, insomnia, lacrimation, pupillary dilation, rhinorrhea, and yawning. In withdrawal from heroin or morphine, symptoms begin in six to eight hours of last use, peak in two to three days, and resolve in seven to ten days. Withdrawal from meperidine peaks in eight to twelve hours of last use and subsides in four to five days.

Opisthorchiasis. A parasite infestation in which worms in the larger bile ducts produce hepatic lesions. Infection is caused by eating uncooked fish.

Oppositional Disorder. A mental disorder that usually begins during late childhood or early adolescence. It is characterized by persistent opposition to authority figures, particularly parents and teachers. This is evidenced by repetitive stubbornness, temper tantrums, procrastination, disobedience, and negativism. It may last for several years therefore precluding academic success and the maintaining of close interpersonal relationships.

Organic Affective Syndrome. *See* Affective Syndrome, Organic.

Organic Brain Syndrome. Those conditions that involve psychological or behavioral abnormalities associated with transient or permanent brain dysfunction caused by specific organic factors. They include anmestic syndrome, delirium, dementia, intoxication, organic delusional syndrome, organic affective syndrome, organic hallucinosis, organic personality syndrome, and withdrawal.

Organic Delusional Syndrome. *See* Delusional Syndrome, Organic.

Organic Hallucinosis. *See* Hallucinosis, Organic.

Organic Mental Disorders. Disorders that are diagnosed by the presence of at least one organic brain syndrome and by the presence of the specific organic factor that is causing the abnormal mental state. Organic factors are diverse and include head trauma, systemic illnesses that affect the brain, toxic agents, primary brain disease, and substance withdrawal.

Organic Personality Syndrome. A mental condition characterized by a distinct personality change that is manifested by apathy, emotional lability, impulsivity, or paranoid ideation. Specific organic causes can be found, the most common being head trauma, neoplasms, and vascular disease.

Oriental Sore. *See* Leishmaniasis.

Oroya Fever. A form of bartonellosis characterized by sudden onset of high fever, extreme pallor, weakness, and anemia. There is also severe muscle and joint pain and headache. Delirium and coma are terminal manifestations.

Osteïtis Deformans. *See* Paget's Disease.

Osteogenesis Imperfecta. A genetic disorder of connective tissue involving the skeleton, ear, joints, ligaments, teeth, sclera, and skin. The cardinal signs are multiple fractures because of narrow and fragile bones, progressive otosclerosis resulting in deafness, kyphoscoliosis, flat feet and joint dislocations because of loose-jointedness, and hypoplasia of the dentine and pulp of the teeth resulting in misshapen, blue-yellow teeth.

Osteomalacia. A disorder of the adult skeleton in which there is defective mineralization. Causes include vitamin D deficiency, underexposure to sunlight, intestinal malabsorption of vitamin D, chronic acidosis, and prolonged anticonvulsant medication therapy. Clinical manifestations include skeletal pain, bone tenderness, muscular weakness, bones fracturing easily, and deformities.

Osteoporosis. The condition in which there is reduction in bone mass sometimes so severe that the skeleton can no longer support the body. Clinical features include frequent fractures of the long bones, back pain, and spine deformity.

Otitis Externa (swimmer's ear). An inflammation of the external auditory canal commonly as a result of furunculosis, bacterial infection, yeasts, and dermatoses. Pain, fever, and lymphadenitis are usual symptoms.

Otitis Media. A middle ear infection. Clinical manifestations include fever, eating problems, irritability, pain, decreased hearing, and bulging tympanic membrane.

Overanxious Disorder. A mental disorder of childhood characterized by extensive worry and anxiety. The child is extremely sensitive, continually worries about his or her abilities and future events, has somatic complaints without physical findings, and demonstrates a need for almost continuous reassurance. The disorder is common and may become chronic, extending into adult life as an anxiety disorder.

P

Paget's Disease (osteitis deformans). A disease of the bone characterized by excessive resorption of bone followed by replacement with coarse-fibered dense disorganized bone cells. Clinical features include swelling or deformity of long bones, gait disturbance, enlargement of the skull, pain in the face, headache, pain in the back and lower extremities, and hearing loss.

Pancreatitis. Inflammation of the pancreas caused by autoenzymatic digestion of the organ. Pancreatic enzymes can also escape into nearby tissues and the peritoneal cavity. Clinical manifestations include abdominal and back pain, nausea and vomiting, ascites, and shock.

Panic Disorder. An anxiety disorder characterized by the occurrence of panic attacks. The attacks are preceded by feelings of apprehension, fear, or doom. Symptoms of the attacks include tachycardia, palpitations, chest pain, trembling, vertigo, hot and cold flashes, and fear of dying or losing control. An attack usually lasts a few minutes, but fear of future attacks may cause the individual to curtail activities in order to avoid being alone if and when a future attack occurs.

Papillon-LeFévre Syndrome. An inherited condition characterized by keratoderma of the palms and soles and premature peridontoclasia. The gingivae become red, swollen, boggy, and bleed easily. Gingivae return to normal when all the permanent teeth are lost.

Paranoid Disorders. Disorders that include paranoia, shared paranoid disorder, and acute paranoid disorder. In all paranoid disorders there are delusions that are persecutory or involve jealousy. The delusions are recurrent and the individual's behavior is consistent with the content of the delusions. There are no other symptoms. PARANOIA is diagnosed when the delusional system has stabilized and lasted for at least six months. A SHARED PARANOID DISORDER (Folie à deux) may develop in a close relationship with another individual who already has persecutory delusions. The delusions are at least partially shared until the relationship is terminated. An ACUTE PARANOID DISORDER is one lasting less than six months. It is the only paranoid disorder that rarely becomes chronic. The other disorders tend to begin in middle or late adult life. Due to the persistence of the delusions, severe marital and social problems frequently result.

Paranoid Personality Disorder. A personality disorder characterized by long-standing patterns of behavior that evidence a lack of trust in and suspiciousness of others. Manifestations include an overconcern with hidden motives, hypervigilance, and a tendency to take offense easily. Individuals with this disorder have difficulty relaxing, are cold and aloof, and avoid close interpersonal relationships.

Paranoid Type, Schizophrenic Disorders. *See* Schizophrenic Disorders, Paranoid Type.

Parkinson's Disease (paralysis agitans). An extrapyramidal syndrome characterized by abnormal gait and involuntary movement. Onset is usually middle to late life, and etiology and mechanism are still unclear. Clinical features include stooped posture, stiff and slow movements, a fixed facial expression, tremor of limbs, and monotonous voice.

Paroxysmal Polyserositis. *See* Mediterranean Fever.

Passive-Aggressive Personality Disorder. A personality disorder characterized by long-standing patterns of behavior that impair both interpersonal relationships and work productivity. It is manifested by persistent indirect and passive expressions of anger. Examples include stubbornness, procrastination, dawdling, obstructionism, and intentional inefficiency.

Pathological Gambling. *See* Gambling, Pathological.

Pedophilia. A psychosexual disorder characterized by sexual excitement being attained through either the fantasy of or actual engagement in sexual activity with children.

Pellagra. A disease of niacin deficiency. Causes include inadequate dietary intake and poor absorption. Clinical features include dermatitis, diarrhea, fatigue, insomnia, apathy, confusion, disorientation, hallucinations, paresthesias, polyneuritis, achlorhydria, glossitis, vaginitis, and general chronic wasting.

Pelvic Inflammatory Disease (PID). An acute infection of the pelvic viscera usually caused by cervicovaginal bacteria such as gonorrhea, and incidence can rise with insertion of an intrauterine contraceptive device (IUD). Clinical manifestations include lower abdominal pain, abnormal vaginal discharge, abnormal menstrual discharge, fever, chills, nausea, adnexal mass, dysuria, and proctitis.

Pendred Syndrome. An inherited disorder consisting of deafness that is usually present at birth and goiter that occurs at puberty. Hypothyroidism may also be present.

Peptic Ulcer. A term referring to upper gastrointestinal ulcerative disorders of unknown etiology associated with the presence of acid-pepsin. The major forms are duodenal and gastric ulcers. Clinical manifestations include epigastric pain occurring characteristically one and one-half to three hours after eating and usually relieved by food or antacids, weight loss, and bleeding resulting in tarry stools and vomiting blood or "coffee-ground" material.

Periarteritis Nodosa (polyarteritis nodosa). A necrotizing inflammation of the medium and small arteries and adjacent veins but not the capillaries. Clinical features include fever, weakness, anorexia, weight loss, myalgia, arthralgia, retinal exudates and hemorrhages, pericarditis, pleuritis, glomerulosclerosis, and mesenteric vasculitis.

Peritonitis. An inflammation of the peritoneal cavity resulting in paralytic ileus, fever, tachycardia, nausea and vomiting, anorexia, and abdominal tenderness with muscle rigidity and rebound tenderness.

Personality, Depressive. *See* Dysthymic Disorder.

Personality Disorder, Antisocial. *See* Antisocial Personality Disorder.

Personality Disorder, Avoidant. *See* Avoidant Personality Disorder.

Personality Disorder, Borderline. *See* Borderline Personality Disorder.

Personality Disorder, Compulsive. *See* Compulsive Personality Disorder.

Personality Disorder, Dependent. *See* Dependent Personality Disorder.

Personality Disorder, Histrionic. *See* Histrionic Personality Disorder.

Personality Disorder, Narcissistic. *See* Narcissistic Personality Disorder.

Personality Disorder, Paranoid. *See* Paranoid Personality Disorder.

Personality Disorder, Passive-Aggressive. *See* Passive-Aggressive Personality Disorder.

Personality Disorders. Disorders manifested when particular personality patterns or traits are incompatible with the successful maintenance of interpersonal relationships or occupational functioning. They are manifested through inflexible and limited patterns of behavior that are usually evidenced in adolescence and persist throughout life.

Personality Disorder, Schizoid. *See* Schizoid Personality Disorder.

Personality, Hysterical. *See* Histrionic Personality Disorder.

Personality Multiple. *See* Multiple Personality.

Personality Syndrome, Organic. *See* Organic Personality Syndrome.

Perthe's Disease. A bone condition of unknown cause consisting of asceptic necrosis of the capital femoral epiphysis. Symptoms include pain, limitation of motion, and swelling.

Pertussis (whooping cough). A bacterial infection, primarily of infants and small children, causing acute bronchitis. Clinical features following a seven- to ten-day incubation period include paroxysmal cough with a prolonged inspiratory stridor ("whooping"), sneezing, fever, rhinorrhea, and anorexia.

Peter Syndrome. An inherited disorder consisting of ocular defects, skeletal anomalies, developmental defects of the gastrointestinal tract and central nervous system, hydro-cephalus, and mental retardation.

Phencyclidine (PCP) Abuse. Characterized by intoxication during greater portions of the day and by episodes of a mixed organic mental disorder or delirium. Interpersonal relationships and work productivity are adversely affected as a direct result of the pattern of use. Neither tolerance or withdrawal syndromes have been evidenced.

Phencyclidine (PCP) Organic Mental Disorders. Disorders that include intoxication, delirium, and a mixed organic mental disorder. Symptoms of INTOXICATION include euphoria, grandiosity, marked anxiety, emotional lability, impulsivity, impaired judgment, ataxia, numbness, diaphoresis, and dysarthria. Intoxication may last up to six hours after use. A DELIRIUM, manifested by alterations in the level of consciousness, may occur within twenty-four hours of use or after recovery from an overdose, and may last for one week. A MIXED ORGANIC MENTAL DIS-ORDER, evidenced by the presence of several organic brain syndromes at one time or a change from one syndrome to another may occur. These include delirium, delusions, and hallucinations.

Phenylketonuria. An inherited liver enzyme deficiency condition characterized by toxic serum levels of phenylalanine. Clinical features appear within a few weeks of birth and include seborrheic eczematous skin rash, irritability, vomiting, seizures, and a "musty" odor. Severe mental retardation results if the condition goes untreated.

Pheochromocytoma. Benign catecholamine-producing tumors of the adrenals causing hypertension. Clinical features include attacks of tremor, weight loss, nervousness, palpitations, heat intolerance, and sweating. Attacks may occur frequently every day or years apart, and may last for a few minutes or for a few hours.

Phimosis. An anomaly of the penis consisting of a narrowing of the preputial opening so that the prepuce cannot be retracted. Urination is often difficult and urine can accumulate underneath the foreskin.

Phobia, Simple. A phobic disorder in which unrealistic fear is limited to a specific object or situation. These may include fear of a particular animal, closed spaces, or height. Simple phobias are common; the onset usually occurs in childhood.

Phobia, Social. A phobic disorder in which unrealistic fear is centered around social situations in which the individual may be observed by others while performing such acts as writing, speaking, eating, or drinking.

Phobic Disorders (Phobic Neuroses). Disorders characterized by persistent fears of a particular object, art, or situation that is not realistically dangerous. Individuals with phobic disorders recognize that their fears are not rational, but their attempts to confront the particular situation produces extreme anxiety. There are resultant changes in life style with varying degrees of self-imposed restrictions in order to avoid either the particular situation or the anticipated anxiety.

Pickwickian Syndrome. A condition of extreme obesity associated with hypoventilation. Somnolence, twitching, cyanosis, periodic respiration, secondary polycythemia, right ventricular hypertrophy and right-sided heart failure with ankle edema, and engorged neck veins may also be present.

Piebaldism. A congenital circumscribed hypomelanosis that resembles vitiligo. The hypomelanosis occurs in areas on the extremities and anterior surface of the thorax. The patients are otherwise healthy.

Pilonidal Cyst. A congenital defect resulting from a faulty coalescence of the ectoderm in the midline over the sacrococcygeal region. Infection can enter through sinus tracts and cause swelling, heat, redness, tenderness, and purulent discharge.

Pink Disease. *See* Acrodynia.

Placenta Accreta. An abnormal adherence of the placenta to the myometrium after delivery of a baby due to lack of decidua basalis between the placental trophoblast and myometrium. Chorionic villi minimally invade the myometrium. Clinical characteristics include retained placenta and hemorrhage when removal is attempted.

Placenta Increta. An abnormal adherence of the placenta to the myometrium after delivery of a baby in which chorionic villi penetrate into the myometrium. Clinical characteristics are the same as for placenta accreta.

Placenta Previa. A condition of pregnancy in which the placenta implants in the lower uterine segment, partially or completely covering the cervical os. The characteristic clinical feature is painless vaginal bleeding unrelated to trauma or unusual activity during the latter half of pregnancy.

Polioencephalitis Hemorrhagica Superioris. *See* Wernicke's disease.

Poliomyelitis. An enteric viral infection that affects the spinal cord and cranial nerves. Infections may result in minor febrile illness, aseptic meningitis, or paralysis. Clinical characteristics depending upon severity include fever, cramping muscle pain, muscle spasms, muscle weakness, and urinary bladder and respiratory dysfunction.

Polyarteritis Nodosa. *See* Periarteritis Nodosa.

Polycystic Ovarian Disease. A condition in which there are enlarged thickened sclerocystic ovaries. Clinical manifestations include amenorrhea, obesity, hirsutism, sterility due to anovulation, and retarded breast development.

Polycystic Renal Disease. A congenital disease characterized by abnormal kidneys, the cortex and medulla of which are covered with thin-walled, spherical cysts that interfere with renal function. Clinical manifestations include flank pain, hematuria, nocturia, calculi, palpable kidneys, hypertension, and progressive renal failure.

Polyhydramnios. An excessive quantity of amniotic fluid for the respective stage of pregnancy. The main clinical feature is excessive size of the uterus. Acute polyhydramnios can result in premature labor and neonatal death.

Polymyositis. A disease of unknown cause that affects the striated muscle and connective tissue. Clinical characteristics include symmetric weakness of proximal limb and trunk muscles and aching muscle pain. Onset is insidious and the disease process is slowly progressive.

Pompe's Disease. A disorder characterized by massive glycogen deposition in the cardiac and skeletal muscles, liver, and central nervous system. Clinical manifestations include impaired cardiac function, cyanosis, dyspnea, tachypnea, restlessness, thickening of the tongue and, muscular hypotonicity.

Porphyrias. A group of diseases associated with inherited or acquired disturbances in heme synthesis. The characteristic features are intermittent attacks of nervous system dysfunction precipitated by barbiturates and resulting in abdominal pain, peripheral neuropathy and mental disturbances, and skin photosensitivity.

Post-Traumatic Stress Disorder. A mental disorder that occurs after an extremely stressful event not usually experienced by most people. The traumatic event is reexperienced by the individual either through recurrent dreams or memories, or by a sudden sensation that the event is recurring. The individual may develop a sleep disturbance, guilt over having survived, and difficulty remembering or concentrating. Reduced involvement and interest in previous activities and feelings of detachment from others may be evidenced. The appearance of symptoms may take place soon after the traumatic event or may be delayed for years.

Potter Syndrome. A congenital bilateral renal agenesis. Other associated conditions include oligohydramnios, prematurity, breech presentation, small size, wide eyes, parrot-beak nose, low-set ears, receding chin, spadelike hands, limb abnormalities, dry wrinkled skin, and pulmonary hypoplasia.

Pott's Disease. A tuberculosis spondylitis. Kyphosis and scoliosis are common. Paraplegia may occur when the upper dorsal or cervical region is affected.

Prader-Willi Syndrome. An inherited disorder characterized by small hands and feet, obesity, hypogenitalism, diabetes mellitus, hypotonia, small stature, and mental retardation.

Preeclampsia-Eclampsia. A condition occurring during pregnancy or in the presence of hydatidiform mole characterized by generalized vasospasm resulting in ischemia and dysfunction of the placenta, liver, kidney, and other organs, and cerebral edema and irritability eventuating in convulsions (eclampsia). The three hallmarks of preeclampsia are hypertension, proteinuria, and edema. Oliguria, visual disturbances, epigastric pain, pulmonary edema, and cyanosis may occur as the condition progresses.

Preexcitation Syndrome. *See* Wolff-Parkinson-White Syndrome.

Primary Degenerative Dementia. *See* Dementia.

Prune-Belly Syndrome (triad syndrome). A congenital disorder consisting of abnormal musculature, cryptorchidism, and urinary tract disorders. Clinical manifestations include urethral obstruction and progressive renal failure.

Pseudocyesis. A condition of imaginary pregnancy that occurs in women who are very anxious about pregnancy.

Clinical manifestations include amenorrhea, weight gain, breast enlargement and secretion, morning nausea, gradual abdominal enlargement, and imagined fetal movements.

Psittacosis. A parasitic disease transmitted to man from birds. Incubation period is seven to fourteen days. Clinical features include chills, fever, headache, pneumonitis with unproductive and often bloody cough, photophobia, myalgia, stiffness of neck and back muscles, lethargy, and disorientation.

Psoriasis. A skin condition with a genetically transmitted predisposition. Clinical features include scaling erythematous papules on the scalp, extensor aspects of the arms and legs, and sites of trauma such as elbows and knees.

Psychogenic Amnesia and Fugue. Dissociative disorders characterized by an inability to remember information about one's own identity. Psychogenic fugue also involves a move to a new physical location and the adoption of a new identity. Both disorders begin abruptly, usually after severe psychosocial stress. They are both rare but are more common during wartime and following natural disasters. There is usually complete recovery.

Psychogenic Pain Disorder. A mental disorder usually characterized by the abrupt onset of severe, persistent pain. The pain is either excessive of what would be expected from physical findings or no organic basis for the pain can be found at all. Psychological needs are expressed through pain, which enables the individual to both obtain support from significant others and avoid particular stressors. The individual has no conscious control of the pain.

Psychopathic Personality. *See* Antisocial Personality Disorder.

Psychotic. A term denoting a loss of ability in reality testing. Perceptions and thoughts may be misinterpreted and external reality misjudged, with evidence to the contrary being discounted. Delusions and hallucinations are manifestations of psychotic behavior. "Psychotic" is used in describing both individual behavior and those disorders in which affected individuals suffer from a loss of ability in reality testing.

Pyknodysostosis. A form of osteosclerosis characterized by delayed closure of the fontanels, separated cranial sutures, and hypoplasia of the terminal phalanges.

Pyloric Stenosis. A congenital disorder of the stomach consisting of an elongated, thickened, cartilaginous, and enlarged pylorus with a severely narrowed lumen. Clinical manifestations include projectile vomiting, constant hunger, small and infrequent stools, weight loss, dehydration, and visible gastric peristaltic waves.

Pyromania. A disorder of impulse control in which the individual is unable to resist impulses to start fires. There is tension before setting fires and a sensation of pleasure or release once the fires have been started.

Q

Q Fever. An acute rickettsial infection transmitted to man by animal products that have been contaminated by tick feces. Incubation period is fourteen to twenty-six days. Clinical manifestations include sudden onset of fever, malaise, headache, weakness, anorexia and pneumonitis with a dry cough, and chest pain.

Quintan Fever. *See* Trench Fever.

R

Rabbit Fever. *See* Tularemia.

Rabies. An acute viral disease of the central nervous system that is transmitted to man in the saliva from the bite of an infected animal. The incubation period can range from ten days to one year. Prodromal symptoms include fever, headache, myalgia, nausea and vomiting, sore throat, a nonproductive cough, and a characteristic paresthesis about the site of entry. The disease progresses with symptoms of agitation, confusion, hallucinations, muscle spasms, combativeness, seizures, hyperesthesia, paralysis of the vocal cords, hydrophobia, and difficulty swallowing with characteristic foaming at the mouth. Coma and respiratory failure precede death.

Rat-Bite Fever. An aerobic bacterial infection transmitted to man from the bite of a rat. Incubation period is one to twenty-two days. Clinical manifestations include a macular rash, arthralgia, arthritis, lymphangitis, relapsing fever, headache, photophobia, and nausea and vomiting.

Raynaud's Disease. A peripheral vascular disorder of unknown cause characterized by arteriospasm induced by cold or stress. Clinical features include cyanosis and pallor of the digits associated with paresthesia, numbness, tingling, and burning. Ulcers and gangrene may ensue necessitating amputation.

Reactive Attachment Disorder of Infancy. A disorder of infancy that is attributed to inadequate emotional bonding and caring. It is characterized by an overall failure to thrive, including delayed development of motor skills, delayed physical growth, and a lack of social and emotional responsiveness appropriate to the infant's age.

Reading Disorder, Developmental. Also known as dyslexia, this disorder is characterized by impaired development of reading skills. Reading is slow, reading comprehension is limited, and oral reading is associated with distortions, additions, and omissions. Skills are significantly below the child's intellectual abilities.

Reifenstein Syndrome. A congenital condition of male pseudohermaphrodites in which there is incomplete masculinization. Clinical manifestations include hypogonadism, feminization, gynecomastia, and sterility.

Reiter's Syndrome. A condition that is characterized by arthritis, urethritis, conjunctivitis, and mucocutaneous lesions. It may result from bacillary dysentery, although the exact cause is unknown. Clinical features include urethritis after sexual exposure followed by arthritis, conjunctivitis, and mucocutaneous lesions that commonly appear on the glans penis, palms, soles of the feet, and in the mouth.

Relapsing Fever. A spirochete infection transmitted from man to man by body lice. Infected ticks may also transmit the disease. Clinical manifestations begin abruptly with rigors, headache, nausea and vomiting, photophobia, muscle and joint pain, high fever that is cyclic, petechial rash, cough, cardiac problems, abdominal tenderness, epistaxes, and hematuria. Three to six days after onset, the attack ends abruptly in a crisis only to recur in seven to ten days.

Residual Type, Schizophrenic Disorders. *See* Schizophrenic Disorders, Residual Type.

Respiratory Distress Syndrome (Hyaline Membrane Disease). An often fatal syndrome of immature infants characterized by immature lungs and atelectasis. It is the result of decreased pulmonary surfactant. Signs and symptoms include expiratory whining or grunting, chest retractions, nasal flaring, tachypnea, cyanosis, hypothermia, and "sandpaper" breath sounds.

Respiratory Distress Syndrome, Adult. *See* Adult Respiratory Distress Syndrome.

Retinitis Pigmentosa. An inherited disorder of the eye characterized by peripheral retinal degeneration resulting in night blindness, optic atrophy, and ring scotoma. Peripheral vision gradually deteriorates until there is only "gun-barrel" vision. Deafness, mutism, mental retardation, and a high-arched palate may be associated with this condition.

Retrobulbar Neuropathy. An eye condition characterized by acute impairment of vision in one or both eyes either simultaneously or successively. The condition may progress to complete blindness, with spontaneous recovery and return of vision after a few days or weeks.

Retrolental Fibroplasia. An eye condition that occurs in premature infants who have received high concentrations of oxygen. Neovascularization results in peripheral clouding of the retina. Retinal detachment occurs with scarring, and complete loss of vision is possible if the condition is not arrested.

Reyes Syndrome. A disease of children characterized by vomiting, progressive central nervous system damage, hypoglycemia, hepatic abnormality, and kidney pathology. Jaundice is characteristically absent. Mortality is approximately 50 percent.

Rheumatoid Arthritis. A chronic systemic disease characterized by inflammatory arthritis of peripheral joints and hematologic pulmonary, neurological, and cardiovascular abnormalities. Clinical manifestations include symmetrical arthritis, rheumatoid nodules over the elbow, splenomegaly, interstitial pulmonary thrombosis, and vasculitis.

Rheumatic Fever. A streptococcal inflammatory disease involving the heart, joints, central nervous system, skin, and subcutaneous tissues. Clinical manifestations include endocarditis producing valvulitis and serious permanent cardiac damage, subcutaneous nodules, migratory polyarthritis, and chorea.

Richardson-Steele Syndrome. A progressive supranuchar palsy characterized by disturbances of balance and gait marked by frequent falls, rigidity of neck and trunk muscles, masking of the face, and reduction in voice volume. Patients eventually become bedfast with severe cervical and truncal rigidity.

Richner-Hanhard Syndrome. An inherited disorder characterized by mental retardation, palmar and plantar hyperkeratosis, and herpetiform corneal ulcers.

Rickets. A condition characterized by defective mineralization in the bones and cartilaginous matrix of the growth plate. Inadequate intake, absorption, or utilization of vitamin D is usually the cause. Clinical manifestations include skeletal deformities, susceptibility to fractures, weakness, and disturbances in growth.

Rickettsialpox. A mild, self-limited febrile condition that is transmitted to man from mice by mites. Clinical characteristics appear seven to ten days after being bitten by the mite and include a skin lesion at the site of the bite, sudden fever with chills, headache, myalgia, anorexia, photophobia, and a papulovesicular rash.

Ritter's Disease (scalded-skin syndrome). A toxic epidermal necrolysis involving formation of flaccid bullae, painful exfoliative erythroderma, and a systemic reaction. Clinical manifestations of systemic involvement include fever, refusal to eat, vomiting, prostration, abdominal distension, and jaundice.

River Blindness. *See* Onchocerciasis.

Rocky Mountain Spotted Fever. An acute febrile illness transmitted to man by tick bites. Clinical characteristics appear after a three- to twelve-day incubation period and include abrupt severe headache, rigor, prostration, myalgia, and high fever. A characteristic petechial rash appears on the extremities and trunk on the fourth day of illness. Delirium, shock, and renal failure occur in severe cases.

Rokitansky-Kuster-Hauser Syndrome. A congenital condition characterized by discrete bilateral hypoplastic uteri and associated with developmental abnormalities of the kidneys and total vaginal agenesis. The main clinical feature is amenorrhea.

Roseola Vaccinosa. A mild, maculopapular rash occurring approximately seven to eleven days after smallpox vaccination.

Rubella (German measles, three-day measles). A viral communicable infection that can cause fetal infection and anomalies if it occurs in women who are in their first trimester of pregnancy. Incubation period after exposure to an infected person is fourteen to twenty-one days. Clinical features include malaise, headache, fever, conjunctivitis, and lymphadenopathy. A rash appears on the forehead and face and spreads to the trunk and extremities and usually lasts for only three days.

Rubeola (measles). An acute viral infection transmitted from person to person via the respiratory route. Incubation period is nine to eleven days after exposure. Clinical features include malaise, high fever, conjunctivitis, photophobia, cough, nasal discharge, koplik spots in the mouth, and a red maculopapular rash that starts on the forehead and spreads down to the feet by the third day. Complications can include pneumonia, myocarditis, and encephalomyelitis.

Rud Syndrome. A congenital disorder characterized by oligophrenia, epilepsy, and ichthyosis. Associated anomalies include dwarfism, partial gigantism, hand and feet defects, nerve defects, hypoplastic teeth, and eye defects.

S

Sadism, Sexual. *See* Sexual Sadism.

Scabies (seven-year itch). A skin disease caused by a burrowing mite that is transmitted from person to person by close bodily contact. Clinical features include a papular or eczematous reaction at the sites of skin infestation and severe itching.

Scalded-Skin Syndrome. *See* Ritter's Syndrome.

Scarlet Fever. A streptococcal pharyngitis in which an erythrogenic toxin is produced. Clinical characteristics include sore throat and a rash that starts at the neck and upper chest and then spreads to the trunk and extremities but does not appear on the palms of the hands or soles of the feet. The tongue is covered by a white coat early in the disease, but this disappears on the fourth or fifth day.

Schistosomiasis (bilharziasis). An infestation of blood flukes transmitted to man by ingesting contaminated water. Clinical manifestations include abdominal pain and diarrhea with or without blood, if the infestation is mainly intestinal. Genitourinary infestations can produce painful micturation, frequency, and hematuria. A characteristic dermatitis commonly called "swimmer's itch" can also develop.

Schizoid Personality Disorder. A personality disorder characterized by long-term patterns of functioning in which the individual demonstrates a lack of warmth or affection for others, indifference to the feelings of others, and difficulty in establishing interpersonal relationships. Individuals with this disorder are socially withdrawn and seclusive, preferring solitary activities.

Schizophrenia, Borderline. *See* Schizotypal Personality Disorder.

Schizophrenia, Latent. *See* Schizotypal Personality Disorder.

Schizophrenia, Simple. *See* Schizotypal Personality Disorder.

Schizophrenic Disorders. A group of mental disorders that usually begin in adolescence or early adulthood. Symptoms include loosening of associations, autistic thinking, disturbances in affect, ambivalence, auditory hallucinations, depersonalization, and disorganized behavior. There is loss of reality testing with disturbances in thought perception, affect, and identity. There are usually residual symptoms after an acute episode; full recovery is uncommon.

Schizophrenic Disorders, Catatonic Type. A schizophrenic disorder that is accompanied by prominent psychomotor disturbances. There may be sudden shifts between periods of stupor and excitement.

Schizophrenic Disorders, Disorganized Type. Also referred to as hebephrenic, this schizophrenic disorder is characterized by extreme impairment and a chronic course. Incoherence, blunted, inappropriate, or silly affect, and withdrawal are predominant.

Schizophrenic Disorders, Paranoid Type. A schizophrenic disorder that is accompanied by delusions or hallucinations that are grandiose or persecutory. There may also be delusional jealousy.

Schizophrenic Disorders, Residual Type. A schizophrenic disorder diagnosed when an individual has had a schizophrenic episode in the past, presents some symptoms of the disorder, but shows no outstanding psychotic features. This is a chronic condition, manifestations of which include social withdrawal, illogical thinking, and loosening of associations.

Schizophrenic Disorders, Undifferentiated Type. A schizophrenic disorder in which the individual exhibits psychotic symptoms such as hallucinations and delusions or disorganized behavior. The symptoms are not, however, typical of any one particular type of schizophrenia.

Schizophreniform Disorder. A psychotic disorder diagnosed when an individual demonstrates symptoms of a schizophrenic disorder, but the duration of the illness is not long enough (i.e., less than six months) to be considered schizophrenic. Individuals with this disorder are more likely to experience an abrupt onset of symptoms and complete recovery.

Schizotypal Personality Disorder. A personality disorder in which interpersonal relationships or employment is adversely affected due to long-term patterns of behavior that include characteristics of schizophrenic disorders, but which are not severe enough to warrant a diagnosis of schizophrenia. There are disturbances in thought, perception, and speech that may be manifested by paranoid ideation, magical thinking, inappropriate affect, ideas of reference, circumstantial speech, and social withdrawal.

Scurvy. A condition of vitamin C deficiency. Clinical characteristics include perifollicular hemorrhages, purpura, hemorrhages into the muscles and joints, bleeding, friable and swollen gums, poor healing of wounds, and emotional lability.

Schilder's Disease. A disease characterized by diffuse demyelination of the central nervous system. Clinical manifestations include cortical blindness and deafness, optic neuritis, spastic hemiplegia, paraparesis, aphasia, and seizures. Dementia and coma may occur before death.

Seckel Syndrome. A congenital condition consisting of facial hypoplasia, prominent nose, microcephaly, joint and skeletal deformities, short stature, and mental retardation.

Separation Anxiety Disorder. A disorder of childhood characterized by intense anxiety when facing separation from significant others or familiar surroundings. The anxiety is excessive and is beyond that which would be expected at the particular stage of development. Symptoms include refusal to go to school, somatic complaints, nightmares, refusal to sleep alone, unrealistic fears of traumatic separations from significant others, and social withdrawal.

Serum Sickness. A systemic immunological disorder that results from the administration of antigenic substances. Symptoms begin seven to twelve days after immunization and include urticaria, fever, myalgia, lymphadenopathy, arthralgia, and arthritis. The disorder is self-limiting usually within ten days.

Seven-Year Itch. *See* Scabies.

Sexual Masochism. A psychosexual disorder characterized by the attainment of sexual excitement through experiencing physical pain or humiliation.

Sexual Sadism. A psychosexual disorder characterized by the attainment of sexual excitement through inflicting physical or psychological pain on another person.

Sheenan's Disease. Pituitary necrosis in postpartum patients due to circulatory collapse associated with maternal hemorrhage. Clinical manifestations may not appear for six to twelve months and may be very gradual. Weight loss, lactation failure, amenorrhea, weakness, cold sensitivity, lethargy, apathy, and loss of libido may occur.

Shigellosis. An acute, self-limited bacterial infection of the intestinal tract spread by contact with objects contaminated with infected feces. After an incubation period of one to two days, fever, abdominal pain, and diarrhea occur. Vomiting, headache, and myalgia may also be present. The stools are green and liquid and contain shreds of mucus and various amounts of blood.

Short Bowel Syndrome. A condition resulting from extensive intestinal resection especially of the ileum and the ileocecal valve. Clinical manifestations include gastric acid hypersecretion resulting in dilution and inactivation of pancreatic enzymes, diarrhea, and inadequate absorption surface resulting in electrolyte imbalance, undernutrition, and dehydration.

SIADH. *See* Syndrome of Inappropriate ADH Secretion.

Sickle Syndromes. Inherited disorders of black people in which sickling of the red blood cell occurs when oxygen tension is reduced. Clinical manifestations include impairment of growth and development, susceptibility to infections, anemia because of increased cell breakdown, episodes of painful crises, and organ damage due to ischemia.

Silo Filler's Disease. An acute interstitial pneumonia that results from the inhalation of nitrogen dioxide from freshly filled silos. Clinical manifestations include immediate cough and dyspnea, followed later by chills, fever, and cyanosis. The disease usually progresses rapidly to death.

Silver Syndrome. A congenital disorder characterized by short stature, hemihypertrophy, and increased gonadotropins. Infants present with low birth weight, a small mandible, and shortened, curved fifth fingers.

Simmond's Disease. *See* Sheehan's Syndrome.

Simple Phobia. *See* Phobia, Simple.

Simple Schizophrenia. *See* Schizotypal Personality Disorder.

Sipple Syndrome (Men II). A multiple endocrine neoplasia consisting of pheochromocytoma, medullary thryoid carcinoma, and parathyroid hyperplasia. Clinical features include thyroid mass, signs of catecholamine excess, and multiple abnormal plasma pathology.

Sjögren's Syndrome. An illness characterized by a decrease in tears and saliva, and chronic arthritis. Patients present with dry eyes that burn, itch, and blur the vision, dry mouth with a decrease in taste acuity, difficulty in swallowing solid foods, dental caries, cracks and fissures at the corners of the mouth, dry nasal mucosa with epistaxis and decreased acuity of smell, and rheumatoid arthritis.

Sleep Terror Disorder. A disorder that most commonly begins during childhood and gradually resolves during adolescence. It is characterized by occurrences of sudden awakening during the night, often accompanied by frightened crying. The episodes occur during the early part of the night, may last up to ten minutes, and are manifested by intense anxiety, disorientation, and an inability to be fully aroused. There is no memory of the occurrence in the morning.

Sleeping Sickness (African trypanosomiasis). A disease caused by a hemoflagellate that is transmitted to man from animals by the tsetse fly. Clinical manifestations include high fever, emaciation, recurrent infections, myocarditis, lymphadenopathy, erythematous nodule at the site of the fly bite, transient areas of painful edema on the hands, feet, and periorbital tissues, and a progressive lethargy, droop, and stupor. Tremors, seizures, and coma precede death.

Sleepwalking Disorder (somnambulism). Usually beginning in childhood, this disorder is characterized by occurrences of walking while sleeping with no later memory of the event. Episodes usually occur during the early part of the night and may last up to one-half hour. During the episode the individual can see and walk around objects but has poor coordination. There is little responsiveness to attempts by others to either communicate with, alter the activities of, or awaken the individual.

Smallpox (variola). A severe contagious viral disease transmitted from man to man by airborne dissemination of infected droplets. Clinical features appear after a seven to seventeen day incubation period and include high fever, myalgia, headache, vomiting, and a characteristic skin eruption of firm papules that progress to vesicles and then to pustules. All lesions at a given time are at the same stage of evolution. After three weeks, scabs and crusts form, which leave scars when healed.

Social Phobia. *See* Phobia, Social.

Sociopathic Personality. *See* Antisocial Personality Disorder.

Sodoku. *See* Rat-Bite Fever.

Somatization Disorder. A mental disorder characterized by seeking medical attention over a period of years for numerous persistent physical complaints for which no organic bases can be found. The disorder is more frequently diagnosed in females, begins before the age of thirty, and is chronic. Psychological needs are converted into physical symptoms that are not under voluntary control. Symptoms include musculoskeletal pain and specific complaints relating to particular major body systems.

Somatoform Disorders. A group of mental disorders characterized by the presence of varied physical complaints for which no organic causes can be found. The symptoms are related to psychological needs and are not controlled voluntarily. The somatoform disorders include conversion disorder, hypochondriasis, psychogenic pain disorder, and somatization disorder.

Somnambulism. *See* Sleepwalking Disorder.

Sparganosis. A tapeworm infection acquired from dogs and cats or by ingesting infected frogs. Clinical manifestations present as painful subcutaneous swellings. Periorbital tissues may be involved with marked palpebral edema and destruction of the globe.

Spina Bifida and Meningomyelocele. A congenital anomaly in which there is a lack of fusion of the laminae of the neural arch of lumbar or sacral vertebrae. Meningomyelocele is present at birth and consists of neural tissue covered by a transparent membrane protruding through the unfused neural arches of the vertebrae. Usually brain stem and cerebellum defects known as Arnold-Chiari malformations are present. Clinical manifestations include denervated bladder, anal sphincter, and limbs. Swallowing difficulty, stridor, and tongue atrophy may also be present.

Spondylitis, Ankylosing. A chronic progressive inflammatory disease involving the articulations of the spine, sacroiliac, hip and shoulder joints, and adjacent soft tissues. Clinical manifestations usually appear between fifteen and forty years and include low back pain, pain in the hips, buttocks, and shoulders, ankylosis of the hip joints, and pain on deep breathing if the thoracic skeleton is involved.

Spondyloepiphyseal Dysplasia. An inherited disorder characterized by fragmented, small, and irregular epiphyses. The infant appears normal at birth, but by mid-childhood lordosis, short extremities and large head become apparent.

Spondylolisthesis. A condition of unknown cause in which there is an anterior displacement of the lumbar vertebra and a bilateral defect in the pars interarticularis. Symptoms may appear in adolescence and include low back pain and increasing lumbar lordosis.

Sporotrichosis. A fungal infection transmitted to man from plants through breaks in the skin. Clinical characteristics include painless red papules at site of entry that later form pustules and ulcerate, and mono- or polyarthritis of elbows, knees, wrists, and ankles.

Spotted Fever (cerebrospinal fever, meningococcemia). A bacterial infection that may be asymptomatic or manifested as an upper respiratory infection or meningococcemia with headache, fever, G.I. symptoms, and a petechial or purpuric rash.

Sprue. A disorder characterized by abnormal small bowel structure resulting in malabsorption and intolerance to the wheat protein, gluten. Clinical features include weight loss, abdominal distention, diarrhea, steatorrhea, anemia, bone pain due to demineralization, compression deformities, and kyphoscoliosis.

Stein-Leventhal Syndrome. A disease characterized by hyper-secretion of androgens by the hyperplastic and leuteinized theca interna of the ovary. The patient presents with a history of irregular menstrual cycles, periods of amenor-rhea, and abnormal bleeding. The ovaries become poly-cystic, ovulation is rare, and sterility and virilism are common.

Stevens-Johnson Syndrome. Erythema multiform exudati-vum (bullosum) characterized by lesions of the skin and mucous membranes, fever, and prostration. The hallmark is an erythematous papular skin lesion that erodes, ulcerates, bleeds, and crusts. Conjunctivitis, photophobia, and corneal erosions may result in blindness. Pulmonary involvement can be present.

Stiff-Man Syndrome. A condition that mimics tetanus but is clinically different. The usual clinical picture is of an adult who has intermittent, progressing to continuous spasms of limb and trunk muscles. The cause is unknown and the condition can last for years.

Still's Disease. A form of juvenile rheumatoid arthritis. Clinical features include intermittent daily spiking fever, polyarthralgias, myalgias, maculopapular rash, pericar-ditis, pneumonitis, sore throat, lymphadenopathy, splenomegaly, and abdominal pain.

Stokes-Adams-Morgagni Syndrome. A cardiac condition characterized by complete atrioventricular block leading to fainting and syncopal attacks. The attacks occur suddenly; the patient turns pale, falls unconscious, and may exhibit clonic movements. Cyanosis, incontinence, and confusion may follow the attack.

Strabismus (squint, walleye, cross-eye, trophia). An im-balance of the extraocular muscles causing a functional loss of vision.

Strachan's Syndrome. A disorder of the peripheral and optic nerves that is characterized by amblyopia, neuropathy, and orogenital dermatitis. Common manifestations include paresthesias of the extremities, painful hyperesthesia of the feet, loss of superficial sensation, ataxia, failing vision, stomatoglossitis, and genital dermatitis.

Straight-Back Syndrome. A condition in which there is loss of concavity of the upper thoracic spine resulting in a decrease of chest diameter. Innocent systolic ejection cardiac murmurs then occur.

Stress Disorder, Post-traumatic. *See* Post-Traumatic Stress Disorder.

Stromal Thecosis (thecomatosis, hyperthecosis). A gynecological condition characterized by diffuse proliferation of ovarian stromal cells with multiple foci of luteinization. Clinical features include progressive virilism, menstrual irregularity followed by oligo- or amenorrhea, obesity, hypertension, and disturbances of glucose metabolism.

Strongyloidiasis. An intestinal worm infestation acquired from penetration of the skin by the larvae. Clinical characteristics include transitory skin eruptions, cough, dypsnea, hemoptysis, and bronchospasm as the worms migrate from the skin through the lungs. In the intestine the infestation causes diarrhea, flatulence, and tenderness.

Sturge-Weber Disease. A neurological disease characterized by hemangiomas on the skin within the area of the trigeminal nerve and venous hemangioma of the leptomeninges. Neurological symptoms occur as progressive destruction of the cortex of the brain and calcium deposits develop. Symptoms include focal seizures on the opposite side of the lesion, transient or permanent paralysis, visual defects, blindness on the affected side, and mental defects.

Stuttering. A disturbance in normal speech patterns evidenced through involuntary hesitancy, repetition, or spasmodic stumbling over particular sounds.

Subaortic Stenosis. *See* Idiopathic Hypertrophic Subaortic Stenosis.

Substance Abuse. The use of a substance to the degree that one is not able to limit use, may be intoxicated for greater portions of the day, or continues to use the substance despite physical problems that continued use aggravates. As a result of the pattern of use, interpersonal relationships and working abilities are adversely affected.

Substance Dependence. Physiological dependence on a particular substance as manifested through tolerance or withdrawal. TOLERANCE is evidenced by the need to take increasingly larger doses of a substance in order to attain the needed effects. WITHDRAWAL is evidenced by symptoms, dependent on the particular substance, that result after decreasing or stopping use.

Sudden Infant Death Syndrome (crib death). The unexpected death of an otherwise well infant whose death cannot be explained by autopsy. Most infants are between ages two to four months and they die at night, unobserved, after having been put to bed in a perfectly well condition. The mechanism of death is unknown.

Summer Grippe (Summer Febrile Illness). A viral upper respiratory infection occurring in the summer and early fall and characterized by headache, sore throat, and anorexia.

Sunstroke. *See* Heat Pyrexia.

Swift's Disease. *See* Acrodynia.

Swimmer's Ear. *See* Otitis Externa.

Swimmer's Itch (cercarial dermatitis). A pruritic, papular eruption caused by the penetration of schistosome blood flukes. Can be acquired both in fresh and salt water.

Swyer Syndrome. A pure XX gonadal dysgenesis. Patients have a female genotype complete with vagina, uterus, and fallopian tubes, but their gonads are streak devoid of germ cells. Clinical manifestations include primary amenorrhea, no breast development, and minimal virilization.

Syndrome of Inappropriate ADH Secretion (SIADH). A disorder characterized by continual release of ADH (antidiuretic hormone) from the pituitary gland that is unrelated to plasma osmolality. The hallmark of SIADH is hyponatremia due to water retention in the presence of urine osmolality higher than that of plasma. Clinical features include weight gain, weakness, lethargy, mental confusion, convulsions, and coma. Edema is rarely evident.

Syphilis. A chronic systemic infection, usually sexually transmitted and caused by a spiral-shaped microorganism. Clinical manifestations occur two to six weeks after exposure and start with a primary lesion(chancre) at the site, which then heals spontaneously. Six weeks later the manifestations of secondary syphilis appear and include skin rash, nontender lymphadenopathy, pustular skin lesions, patchy alopecia, and superficial mucosal erosions of the lips, mouth, and genitals. Late syphilis is characterized by progressive inflammatory disease of the aorta and central nervous system.

Systolic Click-Murmur Syndrome. A cardiac abnormality characterized by excessive mitral valve leaflet tissue. It is usually benign and the patient asymptomatic, but it may lead to significant regurgitation and ventricular dilatation. Clinical manifestations may be present and include arrhythmias and vague chest pain. The main characteristic is a mid or late systolic click.

T

Taeniasis Saginata. An intestinal infestation of beef tapeworms acquired by ingesting undercooked infected beef. Clinical characteristics include weight loss, epigastric pain, diarrhea, and hunger sensations. Movements of the worms at the anus may be felt.

Taussig-Bing Syndrome. A congenital malformation consisting of transposition of the aortic and the pulmonary arteries; the aorta arises from the right ventricle and the pulmonary artery overrides the ventricular septum. There is also ventricular septal defect. The clinical picture includes cyanosis, tachypnea, frequent respiratory infections, decreased exercise tolerance, and poor physical development.

Tay-Sach's Disease. An inborn error of metabolism. The presenting features are developmental delay starting in the third month, progressive neurologic deterioration, macrocephaly, seizures, and retinal cherry-red spots.

Tay Syndrome. A congenital disorder characterized by erythema and scalding at birth, hair abnormalities, and mental and physical retardation.

Teniasis. An intestinal infestation of pork tapeworms acquired by ingesting undercooked pork. Clinical manifestations include muscle pains, diarrhea, fever, and menigoencephalitis.

Testicular Feminizing Syndrome (androgen-insensitivity syndrome). A congenital condition in which the female patient is a gonadal male with active testicular tissue.

Tetanus (lockjaw). An acute disease caused by an exotoxin of an anaerobic bacterium. The disease is often fatal, but those who recover have no residual effects. Clinical characteristics appear two to fifty-six days after the bacteria enter a laceration or puncture wound and include restlessness, irritability, and headache followed by pain and stiffness in the jaw, abdomen, and back, and difficulty swallowing. Rigidity and reflex spasms occur and patients are unable to open their mouths. Laryngospasm and hypoxia may lead to central nervous system damage and death.

Tetralogy of Fallot. A congenital cardiac malformation of the following four characteristics: ventricular septal defect, obstruction to right ventricular outflow, right ventricular hypertrophy, and overriding of the aortic orifice above the ventricular defect. Babies exhibit manifestations such as cyanosis, dyspnea on exertion, retarded growth, clubbing of the nails, and a squatting posture.

Thalassemias. A group of congenital disorders characterized by hypochromic and microcytic red blood cells due to a defect in hemaglobin synthesis. Clinical manifestations include mild anemia, splenomegaly, and icterus. Many patients are asymptomatic.

Thecamatosis. *See* Stromal Thecosis.

Thrombophlebitis. A condition in which there is a clot formation in a vein (usually a leg vein) because of phlebitis or compromised blood flow. Clinical manifestations include pain in the calf of the leg upon dorsiflexion (Homan's sign), swelling of the affected limb, muscle ache, and ankle edema.

Tic Disorder, Chronic Motor. A disorder characterized by involuntary, purposeless, spasmodic muscular contractions. These symptoms may be intense over a period of months. They can be voluntarily controlled for very brief periods.

Tic Disorder, Transient. A disorder that occurs during childhood or adolescence and is characterized by involuntary, purposeless, spasmodic muscular contractions. The most common tics are facial. Symptoms may be voluntarily controlled for a few hours and then reappear. The condition is aggravated by stress.

Thomsen's Disease. An hereditary disease characterized by difficulty in initiating movement and slowness of relaxation. The disease manifestations begin at six to eight years and include myotonia and muscular hypertrophy.

Thrush (oral moniliasis). An oral fungal infection manifested by white, flaky plaques covering all or part of the tongue, lips, and buccal membranes. When removed they leave an inflamed base.

Tietze's Syndrome. A condition characterized by swelling, pain, and tenderness in the upper costochondral cartilages. The onset is often associated with trauma. The joints are swollen and tender but not warm.

Tinea. *See* Dermatophytosis.

Tinea Cruris. A fungal infection affecting the genitocrural areas. Clinical features include erythematous patches with vesiculation, crusting, and scaling.

Tobacco Dependence. An individual is considered to be dependent on tobacco when an attempt to reduce or stop use has been made but the individual is either unsuccessful or experiences withdrawal symptoms. An individual who has a serious physical condition that is aggravated by continued use of tobacco and who persists in its use is also considered to be dependent.

Tobacco Organic Mental Disorder. An organic mental disorder associated with tobacco use. Tobacco withdrawal may be experienced after a sharp decrease or sudden stopping of tobacco use. Symptoms include anxiety, craving for tobacco, difficulty concentrating, headache, irritability, and restlessness. Symptoms peak within twenty-four hours after the last use and gradually decline over a period of up to several weeks.

Tolosa-Hunt Syndrome. An eye disorder of unknown etiology characterized by painful unilateral paralysis of one or more oculomotor nerves. There is acute retro-orbital pain, diplopia, ptosis, and mydriasis.

Tongue-Tie (ankloglossia). A condition in which the lingual frenum extends to the tip of the tongue interfering with its protrusion.

Torticollis (wry neck). A condition in which there is a shortening or contracture of the sternocleidomastoid muscle on one side. The head is tilted toward the affected side and the chin is turned toward the opposite side.

Torulopsis. A fungal infection often resulting in catheter-induced sepsis or endocarditis, gastrointestinal infection, and urinary tract infection in debilitated patients. Clinical manifestations mimic candidiasis.

Tourette's Disorder. A chronic disorder beginning in childhood that is characterized by both motor and vocal tics. The vocal tics may be expressed as barks, coughs, grunts, or yelps. The symptoms, which are aggravated by stress, can be voluntarily controlled for only very brief periods. Neurological abnormalities are found in half of those with the disorder.

Toxic Shock Syndrome. A bacterial infection affecting primarily otherwise healthy young women during their menstrual cycle. A connection with the use of tampons is being investigated. Clinical manifestations include a sudden onset of high fever, vomiting, and diarrhea, with a progression to hypotension and shock. There is an erythematous macular rash that leads to desquamation and peeling of the palms of the hands and soles of the feet.

Toxocariasis (visceral larva migrans). An infestation of ascarids acquired from the intestinal excreta of dogs and cats.

The larvae in the tissues cause hemorrhage, necrosis, and inflammation. The liver, brain, heart, skeletal muscles, and eyes are affected. Clinical manifestations include fever, tender hepatomegaly, skin rash, and recurring pneumonitis. Death may be the result of respiratory failure or cardiac or nervous system involvement.

Toxoplasmosis. A protozoan infestation causing lymphadenopathy, malaise, fever, myalgia, headache, sore throat, maculopapular rash (which is absent from palms and soles), and hepatosplenomegaly. The disease is acquired by ingesting undercooked lamb, pork, and beef, and from cat excreta.

Transient Tic Disorder. *See* Tic Disorder, Transient.

Transsexualism. An uncommon psychosexual disorder in which an individual psychologically identified with one sex but has the physical attributes of the other, resulting in an overwhelming desire to be treated as and to become a member of the other sex.

Transvestism. A psychosexual disorder in which a heterosexual person dresses in clothing of the other sex in order to attain sexual excitement.

Traumatic Neurosis. *See* Post-Traumatic Stress Disorder.

Trematodiasis (liver fluke). An infestation of flukes acquired by eating raw fish or aquatic plants. Dilatation and hypertrophy of the bile ducts is caused by the presence of the flukes. Biliary and circulatory obstruction may be caused with heavy infestations.

Trench Fever (volhynia fever). A rickettsial disease transmitted from man to man by the body louse. Clinical features appear after ten to thirty days of infestation and include headache, relapsing fever, and severe pain in the muscles, bones, and joints.

Trench Mouth (Vincent's stomatitis). An acute necrotizing ulcerative gingivitis caused by malnutrition and poor oral hygiene. Clinical manifestations include tender bleeding gums, fetid breath, gray exudate, and a bad taste in the mouth. Extensive ulceration can result in fever and cervical lymphadenopathy.

Triad Syndrome. *See* Prune-Belly Syndrome.

Trichinosis. An intestinal and tissue infestation by a nematode acquired by ingesting undercooked pork or bear meat. Clinical manifestations appear one to two days after ingestion and include diarrhea, abdominal pain, nausea, prostration, and fever. Muscular invasion of the larvae produces eyelid edema, conjunctivitis, muscle pain, severe weakness, maculopapular rash, myocarditis, polyneuritis, delirium, and coma.

Trichocephaliasis. *See* Trichuriasis.

Trichomoniasis. A protozoan venereal infection manifesting symptoms of vaginitis with profuse creamy leukorrhea or prostatitis, itching, burning, leukorrhea, and urethritis.

Trichostrongyliasis. An intestinal infestation acquired by eating leafy plants that have been contaminated with larvae from the intestines of herbivorous animals. Most infections are asymptomatic, but epigastric distress and anemia may occur.

Trichuriasis (whipworm, trichocephaliasis). An intestinal infestation of worms commonly occurring in the tropics and in areas of poor sanitation. Clinical manifestations include nausea, abdominal pain, diarrhea, and dysentery.

Truncus Arteriosus. A congenital cardiac defect characterized by a single arterial trunk exiting from both ventricles and supplying the systemic, pulmonary, and coronary circulations, and a ventricular septal defect. Clinical manifestations include dyspnea, fatigue, heart failure, recurrent respiratory infections, and poor physical development. Cyanosis is minimal or absent.

Trypanosomiasis. *See* Sleeping Sickness.

Tuberculosis. A necrotizing bacterial infection commonly affecting the lungs; kidneys, bones, lymph nodes, and meninges may also be affected. Port of entry of the bacteria is usually the lungs. Clinical characteristics include localized nodular infiltrations, fibrosis, and cavitation with such manifestations as hemoptysis, pleurisy with effusion, pneumonia, fistula, empyema, enlarged lymph nodes, inflammation of the epididymis and vas deferens, endometritis, tenosynovitis, spondylitis, pericarditis, and meningitis.

Tularemia (rabbit fever, deer-fly fever, Ohara's disease). A bacterial infection transmitted to man from animals by ticks. Clinical manifestations occur three to seven days after the tick bite and include regional lymph node enlargement, lesion at the bite area, fever, and pneumonia.

Turner's Syndrome (a form of gonadal dygenesis). A congenital disorder of females characterized by amenorrhea, sexual infantilism, short stature, and bilateral streak gonads.

Typhoid Fever. An acute systemic salmonella infection acquired by ingestion of contaminated food, water, or milk. Clinical manifestations appear after an incubation period of three to sixty days and include chills, remittent fever, headache, abdominal cramps, rose-spots rash, constipation, and liver and spleen enlargement. Complications can include peritonitis, intestinal hemorrhage, bowel perforation, meningitis, osteomyelitis, arthritis, pyelonephritis, and pneumonia.

Typhus. A severe febrile rickettsial disease transmitted to man by the body louse. Clinical features appear in about seven days and include headache, chills, high fever, prostration, and an irregular macular rash. Spasticity, agitation, stupor, and coma can ensue.

U

Ulcerative Colitis. A chronic inflammatory disease of the large intestine with mucous membranes that are hyperemic and bleed easily. Clinical manifestations include recurrent diarrhea, abdominal pain, rectal bleeding, anorexia, weight loss, malaise, nausea, and vomiting.

Uncinariasis (hook worm, ancylostomiasis). A worm infestation in which the worms enter through the skin, migrate via the blood stream through the lungs to the intestines where they attach to the intestinal mucosa. Clinical manifestations include skin lesions at site of entry, cough, fever, bronchial irritation in the lungs, and symptoms of enteritis and anemia.

Undifferentiated Type, Schizophrenic Disorders. *See* Schizophrenic Disorders, Undifferentiated Type.

Undulant Fever. *See* Brucellosis.

Urethrotrigonitis (the urethral syndrome). An inflammation of unknown cause occurring in the lower urinary tract. Clinical manifestations include severe urinary urgency and a feeling of pressure in the presence of an empty bladder. Otherwise the patient is well.

Usher Syndrome. An inherited disorder characterized by retinitis pigmentosa, nerve deafness, mental retardation, and epilepsy.

V

Vaccinia. A viral disease of the skin acquired from smallpox vaccination. Clinical characteristics include progressive necrosis of the vaccination site with destruction of a large area of skin and underlying structures. Metastatic lesions may also occur. Encephalomyelitis can be a complication.

Valley Fever. *See* Coccidioidomycosis.

Varicella. *See* Chickenpox.

Variola. *See* Smallpox.

Ventricular Septal Defect. A congenital cardiac abnormality consisting of an opening between the left and right ventricles of the heart. Left to right shunting and pulmonary hypertension can result. Clinical manifestations depend upon the size of the defect and include murmur, dyspnea, tachypnea, feeding difficulties, growth retardation, recurrent pulmonary infections, cyanosis, clubbing of the fingernails, polycythemia, and cardiac failure.

Vincent's Stomatitis. *See* Trench Mouth.

Visceral Larva Migrans. *See* Toxocariasis.

Volhynia Fever. *See* Trench Fever.

Von Eulenberg's Disease. Congenital paramyotonia. The characteristic of this abnormality is stiffness, weakness, and paralysis following exposure to cold.

Von Gierke's Disease. An inherited abnormality of glycogen metabolism characterized by hepatomegaly, hypoglycemic seizures, failure to thrive, respiratory infections, bleeding diathesis, "doll-like" facies, eruptive xanthomas, lipemia retinalis, and a greatly enlarged abdomen with a resultant waddling gait.

Von Hippel-Lindau Syndrome (cerebelloretinal hemangioblastomatosis). A congenital neurologic abnormality consisting of a vascular malformation of the retina and cerebellum. Clinical manifestations include progressive loss of vision, cerebellar ataxia, headache, and papilledema.

Von Recklinghausen's Disease. An inherited disease characterized by spots of increased skin pigmentation and multiple neurofibromas. Pigmented spots are irregular, vary in size, and are coffee colored. The tumors are multiple, of various sizes, and rounded or lobulated. This disease is often in association with other anomalies.

Von Willebrand's Disease. An inherited hemorrhagic condition characterized by a prolonged bleeding time and reduced blood clotting factor VIII activity. Clinical manifestations include epistaxis, easy bruising, and prolonged bleeding. Hemarthroses can occur.

Voyeurism. A psychosexual disorder in which sexual excitement is attained through secretly viewing others who are either naked or engaged in sexual activities.

W

Waardenburg's Syndrome. An inherited condition characterized by an appearance of piebaldism, wide bridge of the nose, frontal white blaze of hair, heterochromia iridis, white eyelashes, and deafness.

Wegener's Granulomatosis. A disease of unknown cause characterized by necrotizing vasculitis and granulomatous inflammation affecting the respiratory tract and the kidneys. Clinical features include headache, sinusitis, rhinorrhea, otitis media, fever, arthralgias, anorexia, cough, chest pain, and hemoptysis.

Weil's Syndrome. Severe leptospirosis characterized by jaundice, azotemia, hematuria, anemia, pyremia, epistaxis, hemoptysis, gastrointestinal bleeding, subarachnoid hemorrhage, and persistent fever.

Wermer Syndrome. A disorder comprised of tumors or hyperplasia of the parathyroids, pancreatic islet cells, pituitary, adrenal cortex, and thyroid. The clinical picture is variable depending upon which of the glands is hyperfunctioning. Patients usually present with one of the following: peptic ulcer, hypoglycemia, hypercalcemia and/or nephrocalcinosis, multiple skin lipomas, or pituitary dysfunction complaints such as amenorrhea or visual defects.

Wernicke's Disease (polioencephalitis hemorrhagica superioris). A thiamine-deficiency disease characterized by sixth nerve (ocular) palsy, diplopia, internal strabismus, ataxia of both stance and gait, mental confusion, and polyneuropathy.

Whipworm. *See* Trichuriasis.

Whooping Cough. *See* Pertussis.

Wilm's Tumor (nephroblastoma). A malignant kidney tumor usually occurring in children two to four years old. Clinical manifestations include hematuria, pain, fever, hypertension, and palpable tumor mass.

Wilson's Disease. An inherited disorder characterized by abnormal hepatic excretion of copper, resulting in toxic accumulation in the organs. Clinical manifestations include jaundice, malaise, ascites, spasticity, rigidity, chorea, drooling, dysphagia, and neurosis.

Wilson-Mikity Syndrome. *See* Bubbly-Lung Syndrome.

Wiskott-Aldrich Syndrome. An inherited condition characterized by eczema, thrombocytopenia, and repeated infections. Fatal infections, hemolytic anemia, nephrotic syndrome, and lymphoreticular malignancy can occur.

Withdrawal Syndrome. Symptoms that develop following either a marked decrease or elimination of a substance regularly used that produced physiological intoxication. Manifestations are dependent on the particular substance used; however, most withdrawal symptoms do include anxiety, decreased attention span, irritability, and restlessness. Symptoms may last up to several weeks depending on the substance used.

Wolff-Parkinson-White Syndrome (preexcitation syndrome). A cardiac condition characterized by premature electrical activation of a portion of the ventricular muscle in relation to atrial depolarization. The characteristic clinical manifestation is paroxysmal supraventricular tachycardia.

Woolsorter's Disease. *See* Anthrax.

X—Y—Z

XY Gonadal Dysgenesis (Swyer's syndrome). An inherited condition characterized by gonadal failure, sexual infantilism, and low serum testosterone levels.

Yaws. A chronic infectious disease of childhood caused by treponemes involving skin and bone. Clinical manifestations appear in three to four weeks after inoculation and include an initial pruritic lesion, regional lymphadenopathy, painful papules on the soles of the feet, gummas of the skin and long bones, hyperkeratoses of the soles and palms, osteitis, periostitis, and hydrarthrosis. Destruction of the nose, maxilla, palate, and pharynx occurs in late yaws.

Yellow Fever. An acute viral infection transmitted from man to man by the bite of the mosquito. Clinical manifestations appear after an incubation of three to six days and include sudden onset of headache, dizziness, fever, furred tongue, congestion of the eyes, epistaxis, gingival bleeding followed by remission, and then return of the fever, jaundice, melena, increased epistaxis, and hematemesis.

Zenker's Diverticulum. A pouch in the posterior aspect of the hypopharynx usually affecting elderly men. Clinical manifestations include dysphagia, regurgitation of stagnant food, and nocturnal fits of coughing.

Zollinger-Ellison Syndrome. *See* Gastrinoma.

Zoophilia. A psychosexual disorder in which sexual excitement is attained through the fantasy of or actual engagement in sexual activities with animals.